Printed in the United States of America

10 9 8 7 6 5 4 3 2 1

Library of Congress Cataloging-in-Publication Data is available on file.

Contents

Acknowledgments

The path to getting a book published can be a difficult one. Yet with this book, there were few obstacles on that path, and for good reason. Everyone who had a hand in seeing the book's realization truly believed in it. To those believers I'd like to say thank you: Seth Bauer, editor in chief of *Walking;* Ericka Kostka, associate editor of *Walking,* who also edits *Walking* magazine's "Ramblings" page; Barbara Bowen, who agented the book; Becky Koh, editor at The Lyons Press, who made everything so easy; and Donna Fennessy, who handled the permissions, and who the FBI needs to hire for its missing persons bureau. Most of all, I'd like to acknowledge all the authors who contributed their personal reflections, insights, and lessons about walking to this endeavor. Thank you for proving that walking is more than just what meets the foot.

—John Stark

Introduction

Since *Walking* magazine began more than twelve years ago, we've reserved the last page of each issue for "Ramblings," a reader-written column about the central role that walking plays in our lives. After digging through years of back copies we found many of these columns to be timeless, dealing with issues that touch all of us. Like treasures from a sealed pyramid, we felt these "Ramblings" needed to be on permanent display. So we gathered them into a collection, which we've entitled *The Walker Within*.

Most of these essays were written by our readers, meaning you don't have to be a professional writer to write one, but you *do* have to be a walker. If you're a walker, you're an observer of life, for what is walking but exploring?

While we take pride at *Walking* magazine for teaching the physical and healthful advantages of walking, our readers have been the ones who've so often enlightened us on its mental and spiritual returns. Through the act of walking people who may have thought they didn't have a line of poetry in them can find themselves enjoying a creative endorphin rush. As these "essays" show, walking can clear a path to the heart of an emotion, empowering one with the gift of expression.

Maybe that's because walking affords us an opportunity to disconnect from everything else; to look at life through both ends of the binoculars, to flip-flop perspectives by seeing everyday objects up close, and at the same time, personal issues from a greater and wiser distance. In a society that's become increasingly addicted to not walking, walking's gifts are that much more precious. Inspiration can come from the most commonplace of events: a passing storm, lights in a farmhouse window, a toddling toddler, a startled animal catching your eye as it crosses the road.

How walking expresses itself takes endless forms, as our readers never fail to show us. It can be an extremely public or private act. Whether done by yourself, with friends, or the family pet, walking can be a time to remember, reconnect, let go, or marvel. For some it's a leap for joy; for others, a dance of defiance. Though it may look easy, walking can be the hardest thing to do. And something not to be taken for granted, as those who've lost it will tell you. Walking's blessings have many disguises, changing people's lives when they least expect it.

In addition to the "Ramblings" columns, we felt this was the perfect opportunity to include other walking-related writings that have come our way, and touched us. Many are writings that for lack of space or other reasons we haven't published, but haven't been able to let go of either.

Anyone who works for *Walking* magazine has heard it asked before: "A magazine about walking, what is there to say?" With this book we can defer that question to its authors, who've found the answers along country roads and on city streets, in cemeteries, backyards and beaches, even airplane aisles and prison yards. Each of the almost fifty personal stories we chose for this collection is an original take on what it means to walk, evidence of how complex the humble act of putting one foot in front of the other truly is.

—John Stark, Deputy Editor

Where the Feet Wander, So the Mind

For the Dogs

Lynn Duryee

"I'm taking the dog for a walk!" I shout to my husband or any child in earshot. It certainly was not *my* idea to get a dog. I already had a full-time job, and kids who had tons of homework, and a house I really, *really* wanted to keep clean. But did anyone listen to me? No, they listened to our perky blonde neighbor who runs an animal rescue shelter. She stopped by one afternoon with a big smile and a trembling Border collie. Okay, so the dog *was* cute, and everyone says the breed is smart. "Please, please, pleeeease!" begged my daughters, cradling the skinny, young dog like a newborn. "We'll train him! We'll take care of him! We promise!"

Well, the law doesn't hold a nine-year-old to her promise, and neither should I. The dog was ours for keeps. It didn't take long to find out that whoever said Border collies are smart never met my dog Kelly. True to his heritage, Kelly was ready to round up herds of sheep, acres and acres of them. Unfortunately, sheep are scarce in our urban landscape, so Kelly, no doubt using his little dog brain, substituted cars for sheep. To keep him from chasing every passing car and to restrain him from nipping the backs of the short legs that entered our yard, Kelly and I started to walk.

The truth is, I always liked to walk, but now I have to. It must be genetic encoding for mothers: we can do for others (including dogs) what we could never do for ourselves. He forces me to walk. Every day. No matter if it's hot or cold, wet or dry, if his day was good or bad, the dog is invariably an enthusiastic walking companion. I've never heard this dog make up a single reason to wiggle out of his exercise commitment, and he has a canine way of expressing disapproval if I try to worm out of mine.

When it's time for our walk, I fly out the door, leaving science projects unfinished and cupcakes unmade. "Sorry girls!" I chirp, snatching the leash from its hook. "The dog needs his walk!" If it's a good day, I find myself singing as soon as my feet hit the pavement, skipping to keep up with Kelly's gleeful pace. If it's not such a good day, I mutter curses at my kids or co-workers, and I force myself to keep going until walking works its wonder. So far, I've always come back home, restored, refreshed, and ready to wrap up that science project and bake all those cupcakes.

What happened in those thirty minutes? Magic, that's all. The solace of claiming one small part of the day for my own and the age-old joy of a canine companion.

Walking every day reminds me to notice the subtle changes nature brings: the early daffodils in winter, the lacey blossoms of wild plum in spring, the lushness of summer gardens, the streaked apples of fall. Some mornings I see the sun rising up for a long summer day, other times I'm there when the first star comes out on an early winter night. My dog's thorough patrol of the neighborhood has helped me cultivate gratitude. I appreciate one neighbor for her fragrant daphne, that buds the first of every February. I adore another for her abundant roses that bloom from Mother's Day to Columbus Day. I silently thank the rich matron down the street for not developing the vacant lots on either side of her house, thus allowing all of us to enjoy her oak trees and the view of the mountain beyond. When I see the bent old man sitting in his wheelchair on his porch, I wave (though he never sees me), and think how lucky I am to have my legs, how fortunate I am to return home to my family.

People aren't all we see on our walks. Kelly has a nose for squirrels. He strains at his tether and arches for the treetops, apparently believing if I would only let him off the darn leash, he could scramble to the topmost branch. We have herds of deer, a menace to the gardeners but a thrill to my dog. There's something for each of us.

On many walks, I see nothing at all, so deeply involved am I in solving a problem at work or resolving a conflict in my marriage. I argue with myself, justify my position, shake my head when I imagine my antagonist disagreeing. Often it's not until the last steep climb home that my labored breathing moves to the forefront of my thinking, and the conflict is set aside, at least for a few minutes.

When I'm going out the door, I call out, "I'm taking the dog for a walk!" But what I should really say is, "I'm going out to reclaim a little bit of my soul."

Walking

GREGORY MCNAMEE

olvitur ambulando, Saint Jerome was fond of
saying. To solve a problem, walk around. Walk
until your shoe leather falls off, until no mole-
skin patch in the world can save the tattered rem-
nants of your heels—only walk, walk as only a
human can until the mysteries of the ages unravel
before you.

Jerome had grand ambitions: to convert the world
to a rising faith. Mine have always been smaller: to
get a handle on whatever happens to be on my mind
at a given time, to wrestle a few problems to the
ground. I have solved a few of them—but probably
not enough—by following his advice. I have roamed
across alpine meanders in Germany, blithely enjoying the *Wanderjahre* of youth while my soldier father
awaited the seemingly imminent Soviet attack on
the Fulda Gap. I have walked, over the years, down
much of the length of the Appalachian Trail, dodging black bears and eighteen-wheelers alike in that
battleground of city and country; over desert paths
on the coast of Baja California, once isolated but
now clogged with resort hotels; along soggy byways
through Somerset and Cornwall, where something
of an older Europe endures; across windswept dune-

fields on the Icelandic coast, a landscape that makes it clear why those old Norse myths are both so noble and so terrifying.

When I was a university student in the mid-1970s, I worked over two summers as an archaeological assistant in southern Italy. The small town in which I lived had been noted in antiquity both as the birthplace of the poet Horace and as a pleasant stopover along the Appian Way, the object of our survey; its last claim to fame was as the birthplace of one of Mussolini's field marshalls. Afterward the town had languished, just another whitewashed village in the shadow of the Apennine Mountains, no place for sophisticates. The town was poor, so poor that the residents of nearby towns called their neighbors *indiani*, as if they were a slice of Calcutta transplanted to Europe. For all its poverty it seemed joyful, however, an apparent contradiction that I pondered on many walks through its streets.

The landscape was littered with trails: goatpaths that had been in use since the Neolithic era; footpaths from Roman times, still carefully maintained so that the locals, accustomed to the ebb and flow of European history, could make for the hills at a moment's notice; cobbled lanes that led to lush vineyards, plum orchards, and olive groves; and far on the flatlands below, a modern *autostrada* that spread its black band of asphalt from Milan to the heel of Italy. Aside from the last intrusion, it was all a walker's dream. Indeed, the people of the village, like most rural Mediterraneans, practiced the custom of ambling each fair-weather evening in a continuous loop through the town, a *passeggiatta* that allowed everyone the chance to visit, if only for a moment, with their neighbors. (Were Americans to take up this custom, the rate of criminal violence would surely drop, for it's easier to gun down strangers than people with whom you've passed the time.)

Walking, I learned over those summers, helps sharpen the senses. At a Pleistocene gait, far removed from the jet airliners and fast auto engines that blur our vision of the world, the walker makes out the shapes of things, learns to distinguish the differences between look-alike plants, to separate out the churring of myriad insects and the whirring of birds—and even to solve a few puzzles. Sometimes the pedestrian's senses can even become too sharp. One early morning while walking among olive orchards that lined a small river, I had the strange perception that I could see straight through the now-shaking trees, that their atoms had somehow disincorporated or that I had suddenly attained X-ray vision like Superman. A few seconds passed until I noticed that the ground below me had momentarily become rubbery. Only then did I realize that I was witnessing an earthquake, that my small corner of the world had indeed flown apart for an instant.

Much of the walking I did in southern Italy was far less revealing. My daily work involved lugging a theodolite across newly plowed fields, hopping among clods of dirt two feet across. The deep plows turned up soil two meters deep, so that buried artifacts from ancient times—bits of pottery or tile, say, or the occasional piece of lead pipe—would be dredged up to the surface. Whenever our team encountered a scatter of such artifacts, we would measure the area, plot it on Italian artillery maps of only nodding accuracy, and then move on in search of the next scatter. It was exhausting work, more suited to oxen than to humans; even the farmers avoided walking in those churned-up fields. In two summers, by my estimate, we traversed twelve hundred miles of black soil, a part of Italy that very few visitors ever see, or would ever want to see.

I solved a career problem in walking those fields. Walkers cannot help but think, after all, if only to distract from sore backs and aching feet. I decided that the glamorous world of archaeology was not to be my profession; the slogging was just too hard. Instead, I became an editor, and then a writer, making a run for unplowed hills whenever the wanderlust became too much to handle.

Nearly two decades later, I find myself spending long stretches of time roaming the deserts and mountains of the Southwest. To live in the desert requires a certain kind of madness—that specific disease of dogs and the English—that is epidemic out this way. To wander off into that desert, alone or in company, is to test the very limits of one's endurance and to tempt the end of one's tenure on this otherwise green planet.

Such ventures make us human. Or, better: it is the walking itself that makes us human, that defines our nature. Our ability to raise ourselves on two feet and not fall over while moving distinguishes us from all other animal species. Only as a consequence of that ability could our brain cases expand enough to allow us to hold the thoughts we have since had, for good or ill. Only then did our laryngeal tract, tugged downward thanks to our newly erect posture, expand so that we could form speech. Thus most babies walk before they talk, and stop crying when they are rocked back and forth, a rhythm that emulates walking.

We were made to wander afoot—read Roy Lewis's subtly hilarious novel *The Evolution Man* for the evidence—and we were made to keep moving. When we settle down, it seems, we tend as a species to become nastier rather than more civilized: the Mongol hordes notwithstanding, nomadic peoples do not loll about inventing secret-police organizations, atomic weapons, and taxes.

Idle feet, it turns out, are the devil's real workshop.

Solvitur ambulando. It is solved by walking around. Walk on quietly, for, as the peripatetic American poet Marianne Moore once observed, "The deepest feeling always shows itself in silence."

Just walk on.

The Walking Bubble

The bubble burst, I think, during the chorus of "Under the Boardwalk."

I was in sport-walking mode, tape player harnessed to my hips, cutting through a highly trafficked street in Providence, R.I., where I live. Stride, stride, smooth as silk, but then that chorus slid through the earphones:

Under the boardWALK

Was that a shoo-bop, slide-step I just did? Nah.

We'll be havin' some fun,
Under the boardWALK

Whoa. That was a shoo-bop, slide-step, topped off by a little curb-jumping jive. I looked around. Pedestrians swirled around—students, mothers, toddlers. Had they witnessed this little show? Did they see a woman in black tights and T-shirt dance past them? What kind of fool was I? And how long had I been doing this?

I spent the next 2 miles reviewing my walking life. I'd been doing this, I realized, for years. Fifteen years ago I spent a collegiate summer in Washington, D.C., and walked a mile each day to work. To fill the time, I worked on my mediocre singing skills. I picked a Paul Simon tune that fit into my narrow vocal range and practiced it every day. For six weeks I sang that same song. Six weeks. Thirty round-trips. And at least 200 fortissimo renditions of "American Tune."

As a working person, I'd use the time to rehearse: arguments I needed to have with my boss, arguments I needed to have with my boyfriend. Recently I had to give a long speech, so I took a walk and made it up on the road. I gave the whole speech aloud, complete with sweeps of arms, accents, and eye contact with my imaginary audience.

All these walks took place in congested areas. I walked past people, storefronts, outdoor cafes, and not once did I think how ridiculous I must have looked. Then it came to me: I'd been in a Walking Bubble.

The Bubble: that same psychological barrier that protects a political candidate from real people, that protects you from fear when you get in a New York City cab, and that had protected me from public humiliation while I walked.

The Walking Bubble. Of course. A Bubble can only form around a person if she is mentally divorced from her physical presence. There's no Running Bubble, because you're going too fast and breathing too hard. No Cycling or Rollerblading Bubble—too much technical challenge. No Archery Bubble, and we can just be grateful for that and move on.

The Walking Bubble. It was the perfect shield. I thought about friends who had stopped me and said, "I saw you walking the other day," and then paused, waiting for me to say something like, "Oh, did you hear me singing?" I'd said nothing, though, and they moved on in their lives and put a mental checkmark near my name. She talks to herself. She dances on city streets. Don't invite her to our next barbecue.

Well, what's done is done. My Bubble is gone, and I'll be walking a little more acceptably now, in the cold air of self-consciousness. Sure, I mourn the loss of my lunacy a little. Wouldn't you? But you're not sure if you've ever been in the Bubble, are you? Don't think too hard. You don't want to pop it before you have to. Just put on the earphones and glide.

The Drum Major in Her Own Parade

Lynn Setzer

'm sitting here at my keyboard in a state of mild euphoria. Why? I just returned from my morning walk with John Philip Sousa.

I learned about the power of walking—and a good Sousa march—a million years ago when I was in high school. A member of the band, I'd go out every day to march during our third period class. Our town was small, rather like the one Thornton Wilder wrote about in *Our Town;* the residents and shopkeepers would step outside on their porches and under their awnings to watch with pride as our little band drilled through the town.

As we marched through the tree-lined streets, we'd play our high school's fight song interspersed with rousing Sousa marches as well as other military tunes. Rum-pum-diddle-diddles played by the percussion section punctuated the relative silence between songs. And because the percussion section was composed of a group of rowdy boys, the tempo was often quite lively. We loved it.

Our band director was adamant that as much of that 50-minute period be used for marching as possible, so we hustled to be in formation just as the tardy bell was ringing. He generally gave us only two minutes at the end of the period to put away our instruments, find our books, and be off to our next round of classes.

The net effect of all of this marching was twofold: I dropped about 10 pounds of adolescent weight without hardly knowing how it happened. I also developed an ability to hear march music in my head any time I went out walking.

Today when I go out for a walk it's impossible for me *not* to hear the music of Sousa. The music starts quietly enough, often with *Colonel Bogey,* better known as the theme from *Bridge on the River Kwai.* Once I'm warmed up, the tunes switch to *Washington Post, Semper Fidelis,* and *El Capitan.* I hear *Anchors Aweigh, National Emblem March,* and *American Patrol* and my stride begins to lengthen. Soon I'm hustling right along, arms pumping and light on my feet, about to take off into the wild blue yonder or land on the shores of Tripoli.

By the time I hear the *Stars and Stripes Forever,* a 150 piece marching band is playing in my head, complete with all of the parts, from the piccolos to the baritones, and all of the clarinets and cornets in between. Absolutely taken away by the music, I imagine fireworks exploding over my head. It's a serious aerobic workout I'm enjoying, as the drum major in my own parade. I'm always surprised that the rest of the neighborhood hasn't come out to hear the music.

When the parade comes to an end—when I arrive at the sidewalk to my house—I am refreshed and ready to take on the world. And I have to tell you, today's concerns, as confounding as they may be some days, beat the heck out of Algebra II.

Walking the Yard

Scott Breeze

I have spent 25-odd years in and out of a dozen or so prisons. Don't ask why, it's considered rude. In each of those prisons men found ways to stay fit, alleviate stress, and maintain sanity through exercise. They exercised in all the traditional ways: sports, running, calisthenics, weights. They also exercised in non-traditional ways: yoga, martial arts, ingenious variations of substitute weights like buckets of sand or water, even push-ups with a guy sitting on your back. Once, I heard about a con who did 7½ years in a 4 × 4 × 4 ft. box but came out relatively fit.

One common thread runs through every con's fitness routine, though: they walk. Whether alone or with one or more "walkies" or "road-dogs" they all walk. Maybe walking the ever present path in the exercise yard provides some subconscious need to feel a sense of freedom, the ability to roam. Being pent up in a 6 ft. × 8 ft. cell 23 hours a day is an unnatural state for humans; as is being unable to walk 40 ft. in any direction without stopping for someone to unlock a door. Walking that well-worn path out in the yard imbues one with an artificial sense of space and travel that is necessary for mental balance. The worst years I ever did while incarcerated were those times when I was unable to take my daily walks. Worse yet were those times when I had to wear shackles that shortened my stride to 18 inches. It's maddening, try it sometime.

The paths in the exercise yards are always the same. They vary in length but always snake along the full fence-line, allowing an inmate to get as close as he can to the security perimeter without getting shot at. They are just wide enough for two to walk abreast, which is usually the biggest crowd you can gather without attracting attention. The paths are worn smooth of most stones or grass by innumerable footsteps over the decades. I've been to prisons over 100 years old that had had their path in the same place since the first convict stepped out onto the yard. Convicts always know how long the walk will be. "How many laps is a mile?" the new guy asks. "Three times around is a mile," the old-timer answers.

I have been in institutions so bereft of activities for the prisoners that walking was the major form of entertainment. Men in solitary confinement will walk up and back for hours in their cells, some like automatons, some like caged tigers. But they walk. After a facility-wide lockdown of several days the most common theme of conversation is "Man, it feels good to walk around!" A good long walk is always in the top ten on the "List of Things I'll Do When I Get Out."

A walk around the yard or the range or tier catwalk can give one a sense of personal space in an environment designed to limit that space. A walk can provide needed privacy for a conversation with a confidant. It can provide the mind space for introspection, a necessity for rehabilitation. I have walked the Appalachian Trail, the galleries of the Smithsonian, my hometown sidewalks and never left the confines of my cell.

Walkers run the full spectrum from serious speed walkers who fly around the yard in their sweats, elbows pumping, hips swaying, to the amblers who mosey along for hours, hands in pockets. Me, I tend to fall somewhere in between the two extremes.

At most institutions the security staff encourages everyone to walk. Not for any concern for your fitness but to keep trouble at bay by discouraging loitering. "Walk and talk! Walk and talk!" rang in my ears for four years at a facility south of Washington, DC. No one could stop to talk to anyone else without attracting the attention of the guards. The result was that the whole facility took on the appearance of some giant disturbed anthill and the guards couldn't keep track of anyone.

Once, in a movie about a Turkish prison, there was a scene where all the insane prisoners were made to march around and around in a big circle all the time. Walking was the last semblance of normalcy in their lives. Walking was something so primal even the incurably mad could identify with it. In the Bataan Death March it was walk or die for prisoners. Stories from the gulags and concentration camps of history are full of references to walking, mostly to stay sane or alive. It strikes me as peculiar that the one people in the world with the least amount of freedom walk so much. It's universal. Check for it the next time you drive past a prison or watch a prison movie. Everyone's walking somewhere—or nowhere.

With 1.8 million people incarcerated in this country I suppose after they are all paroled (85% will be), we will have a nation of walkers. Out of nearly 2 million walking ex-cons do you suppose there's one gold medal Olympian, one David Livingstone, one Neil Armstrong? Maybe we'll be redeemed yet. I'd walk a mile to see that.

Walking and Writing at the Same Time

CLINT KELLY

I am an adventure novelist, therefore I walk.
I walk to unknot a plot.
To bring a recalcitrant character to her senses.

To find beginnings and endings and middles which usually hang out on busy street corners, hog two seats on the bus, or park plumply on park benches along my customary route.

I walk to find the perfect name for a character. Jigs Wiggins. Royce Blankenship. Mags O'Connor. Gretchen the Great Dane. All were met on my appointed rounds. These imaginary ones walked along with me. One stepped gingerly; another slouched dejectedly; a third skipped with abandon. The dog bounded after me with the occasional slap of a moist tongue the size of a chunky chihuahua.

In my walking travels, I find weather. Not simply rain or shine, but drippy, snappish, fleecy, and ominous. Clouds big as bungalows. Hail the weight— and wallop—of falling walnuts. Mist fine as snail sneeze. Sunsets the color of mango and watermelon. The weather of my walks becomes the weather of my plots.

Headed into the wind, I find lots of useful items coming at me. Gust-whipped leaves, a yellow polka-dotted ball thrown from an unseen hand, one skate-boarder lean as a picket slat who used me to execute a magical maneuver that I swear was physically impossible.

All stew bits for my pot of simmering story lines.

But what walking does best of all is take me to the scene of the adventure-in-progress and drop me off like some erstwhile time traveler in a fantastic place or an incredible era.

Step lively and I'll show you what I mean. Down here a mile or so from my house at the end of Olympic View Drive, the road dips steeply into Another World 10,000 miles removed from My Regular World. Here lies Likouala Swamp—55,000 square miles of largely uncharted marsh and dense jungle rain forest. In its dark and murky vastness dwells *mokele-mbembe,* a prehistoric monster which pygmy eyewitnesses say leaves a six-and-a-half-foot swath of trampled vegetation wherever it chooses to drag its tail through the reedy river muck.

In the opposite direction, two blocks and a Lutheran children's home over, is legendary Mt. Ararat, the 17,000-foot-tall volcanic resting place of Noah's Ark. I have been there with climbers, grappling hooks, and high altitude rescue choppers pulling off the most hair-raising escape since Indiana Jones last pulled his fat from the fire. You should have seen the eruption at the corner of Dogwood Boulevard and 50th Street. The neighbors tracked in lava for a week.

One of my favorite destinations is a patch of real estate somewhere along the California/Nevada border. It's a tiny backwater populated with humanity made strange by the quest for gold, solitude, and anonymity. It's home to a new adventure romance series I'm looking to deal.

But to get it fixed in my mind, to taste the grit of it, hear the suspicions in it, sweat the scorching heat of it, I need to walk around it. Feel the up and down of it in my thighs. Suck the fragrance of it into my lungs. Observe the doings of its denizens with my own two eyes.

And so I walk it off. Highland Drive to 54th. Fifty-fourth to Dogwood. Dogwood to Elm. Elm to home. The last time I laced up it was for close encounters with Sarg and Kelli and Spence and Faye, inhabitants of "Al and Sal's Bait Place," "Finch's Hardware and Feed," and "Turquoise Bill's Restaurant and Lounge." Especially interesting since that part of my neighborhood isn't even zoned commercial.

It's all in my mind. Walking lets it out so I can play.

Should you encounter me on my walks, I might be muttering to myself. Testing dialogue. Forging emotional response. Picking sides. Listening for clues to character motivation. Rummaging through an old trunk or two, deciding which baggage best goes with two-fisted Leo Slugitt, the ex-merchant seaman, and which with Kathleen Snow, the dazzling serving girl at Gadsby's Tavern.

Occasionally, you'll see me punch the air or give a whoop of glee. Those are moments of what I like to call my "breakthroughs." When suddenly I know how the boys trapped on a rooftop with no escape will survive the evil police commander sent to shoot them. When the means of stopping the previously unstoppable creature is revealed with all the clarity of a moonlit night. When a dark character finds unexpected compassion and acceptance though what he deserves is destruction.

It is then that I tend to quicken my pace.

"Walk and be happy, walk and be healthy," counseled another novelist, Charles Dickens. Why he did not add, "Walk and be published," I do not know. Perhaps he was too busy getting Oliver Twist out of one jam, or putting Scrooge into another, to concern himself with such pronouncements. But it would not surprise me in the least if one day he had donned his hat, hefted his walking stick, announced to the Dickens household, "I'm going for a walk," and did not return until *A Tale of Two Cities* was pretty well fleshed out.

Show me a dedicated novelist and I'll show you a diehard walker.

Let Us Walk

SISTER JOSEPHINE PALMERI

O h, no," I sighed inwardly as I started to flick off classroom lights, book bag in hand. Laura was at the door. "Sister Jo, can I talk to you? I mean, like . . . do you have time?"

I loved Laura. But today I needed a brisk walk after school. I had taught seven high school classes, full force, gung ho. All day the blue sky and radiant autumn leaves had beckoned from my windows.

I've always been an avid walker, but lately I had been staying quite late after school to grade tests and prepare lesson plans. Just last night I had given myself a pep talk: "You're missing autumn. Walk. Fresh air will get the chalk dust out of your lungs. Do schoolwork at night." I promised myself that today I would walk.

But then there were the students who needed me. Like Laura. Her troubled face left me no choice. "I always have time for you, hon," I smiled.

We sat in the empty classroom as she described her Dad's drinking problem and the havoc it was wreaking at home. I listened, handing her a tissue, trying not to glance out the window to where the janitor was mowing the lawn. The fragrance of freshly cut grass wafted in. I did my best to focus on

Laura. After a long time, she got up to leave. "I know you can't do anything about it, Sister, but thanks for listening." I promised to pray for her and gave her a hug.

I got home just in time for chapel. I knew I had done the right thing, but my feet didn't—they kept tapping with pent-up energy. Then it dawned on me: Why hadn't I taken Laura out walking with me?

The next day was just as beautiful. "I will walk today!" I declared. But at 3 p.m., Jack was at the door.

"Hi. Can I talk to you about something?"

"Sure," I answered. "But it's such a nice day. Want to go for a walk?" We circled a nearby lake and talked about working with emotionally disturbed children, his goal. After an hour, we headed back for school.

On Laura's next visit, she too accepted my invitation to walk. I had a surprise for her. Another student, Tom, had given me brochures from Alateen, a support group for children of alcoholics. "Tom said to tell you his Dad has the same problem, Laura, and he can drive you to the next Alateen meeting, if you like." I shared some coping techniques Tom had learned. Laura was consoled to find she wasn't the only teen with an alcoholic parent. Plus, she'd gotten some exercise.

"I really feel better, Sister. Thank you!"

And so it became a pattern. Whoever came to chat after school was invited to walk with me. One drizzly, cold day Dennis appeared after Scripture class. Could we discuss questions he had about the Bible? No, he didn't mind walking. As we moved briskly around the lake, I marveled at this young man's insight into the spiritual world. Our walk ended with hot chocolate in the convent kitchen.

Sure, not every after-school chat calls for a walk. I don't do blizzards or tornado watches. And when a tearful kid really needs to spill her guts in private, we use the wooden desks in a quiet classroom, with a tissue box close at hand.

But whenever we can, we walk. In the steady stride, inhale-and-exhale rhythm, with fresh oxygen flowing to the brain, these kids find release from the pressures and frustration they face every day. And so do I.

Nature and Place

Just Walkin' in the Rain

Violeta Balhas

Out on this country road in Southern Australia, there is no shelter, and I squint to keep the rain out of my eyes. If Papa, a podiatrist, could see me, he'd berate me: He's given me custom-made foot supports for all of my walking shoes, and here I am sloshing about in my extra-large easy-to-remove Wellies.

A good Samaritan in an infinitely warm and comfortable-looking car pulls up alongside me.

"Are you okay? Do you need a lift?"

I smile apologetically.

"No thanks. I'm just out for my walk."

She displays the unconvinced smile usually reserved for children trying to explain their abstract drawings, and then drives off.

I had made my resolution to start walking in the spring, when the skies cleared briefly and I had some hope that summer was on its way. But the skies were traitorous. One day, as I was getting ready to go out for my walk, I saw the clouds in the distance fraying at the edges with rain.

"Weather's turning," I said to my husband. "What do you reckon? Should I go for my walk?"

"It's up to you," he said.

I remembered my resolution and looked at my walking shoes, which would not fare well in a downpour. Wellington boots? In my family, we all own a pair. Australian country folk know the wisdom of wearing boots outside when spring awakens the snakes: My children aren't allowed out in the long grass without them. You won't get a good workout with them on, reasoned half my brain. It's not worth it; stay inside. But the other half of my brain teased: It'll be fun. Remember how it used to be?

My mother had taught me to love the rain. She had married young, and because she could bear children, she was expected to put away childish things. But she just couldn't resist the rain. One of Mama's friends, who was her neighbor when she was a newly-wed, would always look out the window toward Mama's house when the rain would start, saying to herself, "Let's see what excuse Neli's found to go out in the rain this time." If there were a few items on the clothesline, they'd be brought in one at a time.

I remember one humid summer day when the skies had cracked open, spilling water onto concrete so hot that the raindrops made it sizzle. Mama had rushed into the living room where I was watching television and said, "Quick! Put your bathing suit on!" I ran and played outside until the downpour stopped, despite tut-tutting neighbors peeking through their curtains.

I also remember seeing *Singin' in the Rain* in an ancient theater that showed old movies. Enchanted, I smiled at the face of an absolutely besotted man celebrating his love out in the rain—and I fell in love. Gene Kelly loved the rain, and I knew that if I'd been Debbie Reynolds, I'd be out there leaping and splashing around in it with him.

So when I looked at my Wellies on that rainy day, I thought not just about getting fit, but about the child I'd been. I pulled boots and raincoat on and joyously stepped outside.

A Christmas Walk

David Updike

In recent years, I have found Christmas at my mother's house overwhelming. I wake not to the aching euphoria of childhood, but rather to a dull premonition that this is just the beginning of a long, exhausting day. As the house slowly fills with family and friends, and everyone starts doing something—cooking and cleaning and polishing silver—I can never seem to make myself useful. I end up lighting a fire and sitting before it in a kind of Christmas funk. Time seems to pass at half its normal speed until, finally, it is time to have a glass of sherry and open presents—a ritual I gladly partake of—and by the time it is over I begin to feel in the Christmas spirit.

But, still, the turkey is not cooked, nor the potatoes mashed, nor the last of the guests arrived, and there is another hour or two of loitering—eating dates and figs and cracking nuts, downing another glass of sherry—before we are all finally ready to eat. Grace is said, followed by wine, cranberries, turkey, squash, potatoes, peas, a joke or two with my Great Aunt Mae, a puff on my younger sister's cigarette, laughter, more wine, seconds, clear the table (my role, at last) and finally, we are ready for dessert. Pie.

"Shall we take a walk, first?" someone mercifully proposes, as they do every year, and this, it seems, is the moment everyone has been waiting for. Like a dam that is ready to burst, we pull on our coats and hats, release the barking dogs, and spill out into the dull, warmish overcast of this particular snowless Christmas. Outside, everything is still, and in this somber, marshy landscape, shades of rust and gray and brown, we all seem wonderfully animate, alive.

We follow the dogs over the bridge and then along the road that bends across the marsh—a broad, flat plain of tawny, matted grass that stretches away toward the sea. Acting as emissaries, go-betweens between the world of nature and human beings, the dogs forge ahead and then return, tails wagging, with the good news that the coast is clear. Along the road our numbers distend into little clumps of conversation, and from the edge of the marsh we pluck long, thin reeds with tassles on the end, and hold them high like flags, or brandish them like swords.

There is something imposing about the sight of us all, as we possess, en masse, a kind of tribal clout, like a gentle band of brigands, or a tiny familial army daring the neighbors to come out and take a look. Filled with wine and food, we are happy and giddy, and when we reach the big white gate that says "Private Property," someone pushes it open and we recklessly continue.

We follow the path that leads to the edge of the field which, in turn, stretches toward the horizon and, in the distance, yields to the faint blue edge of the sea. And that, perhaps, is what we have come in search of, because when we were halfway across it our momentum begins to wane, and even the dogs begin to sniff back in the other direction, toward the house, where there is fire and food. But our walk has served its purpose, and for me somehow unraveled the tangle of the day and made it all whole. We have been out in our natural element, breathed fresh air, and seen that nature, in its coy and enigmatic way, treats Christmas much like any other day. We have paraded ourselves before the world, man and beast alike, and thus celebrated our renewed and mysterious presence here on earth.

A Jar in Tennessee

Michael Finley

You know those microcassette recorders that cost $29? I buy them not quite like candy, but often enough that there are several around the house. They are great for taking notes when out walking. Sometimes people see you and think you are schizophrenic, talking to your hand, but that is a small price to pay, in my mind, for being able to "write" on the fly.

Imagine, it is a beautiful fall morning, and I am walking my big standard poodle Beauregard at Crosby Farm Nature Area, alongside the Mississippi River in Saint Paul. It is an undeveloped park with lots of paths cutting through the trees along the shore. A perfect place for a scofflaw to let his dog run wild for a few minutes.

And I have the microcassette machine in my pocket, a generic blister-pack Sony. The morning is gorgeous, with newfallen leaves ankle-deep, and white vapor rising from the river. Once, a four-point deer pokes his head into a clearing.

My dog begs me to chase him. It's his favorite game, a role reversal because chasing others is the center of his life otherwise. But I'm game, and I chug along for a hundred yards with him. We take several switchbacks, going deeper into the trees. When we arrive at the riverbank, I feel in my pocket for the recorder. It's gone.

You know how when something is gone you check every pocket eleven times to make sure it's gone? Well, this was gone. I figure I either dropped it when I made my last note, or it fell out of my pocket during the chase. So I begin backtracking. The dog wants me to chase him some more, but my mood is rapidly darkening and I decline.

Leaves have been falling in large numbers, so the ground is covered with brown shapes and jagged shadows, all of which look like my little machine. I begin calculating in my mind the loss of the unit—maybe $40. Besides, they wear out quickly because you are always dropping them and knocking them on tabletops. I look everywhere I walked—about a two-mile distance—for the little machine. No luck.

I am nearly reconciled to the loss when I spot it, lying on a patch of bare dirt. The battery and tape compartments are both sprung open, and the tape and batteries lay splayed out on the ground, as if a squirrel or crow have given some thought to taking them home, and then said, nah.

I pop the machine back together and push the play button, still ready for the worst, a dead unit. But instead I hear my own voice. I am talking about São Paulo, Brazil, which I visited on business two weeks before. On the tape, I am sitting in a bus on a smoggy artery heading out of town, talking to myself about the beggars I see crouched by the highway signs, and the advertising, with the nearly naked models, and the infinite pastel rows of high-rise apartment buildings.

And now I am standing in a clearing in the forest, 7000 miles away, hearing my high, sped-up voice. The woods are so quiet that this little machine and its tinny little speaker ring clear through the air. Nearby birds, hearing my recorded chatter and finding it suspicious, take wing and flap away to a safer roost.

If you have ever stood between two mirrors and seen the illusion of infinite regression in them, you have an idea what I am feeling, addressing myself electronically from a place so different and so far away.

And if that was not stunning enough, I flip the tape over—I do not want to tape over this interesting travelogue—and there is my daughter's voice, talking to a caller on the phone. I re-use my answering machine tapes in my hand recorder, and this tape is perhaps five years old, when my little girl was eight. Her voice sounds so clear, so young and lovely. I forgot what she sounded like then. I can't tape over this either.

The dog, meanwhile, is standing there looking at me with that panting grin dogs wear when they are in their element to the hilt. But the look on his face just now is all wonderment and admiration. He "understands" very little that I do, but this latest trick, picking something up in the woods and having it talk to me in my own voice, well, this just takes the cake.

Insurance company executive and poet Wallace Stevens once wrote a simple poem called "A Jar in Tennessee," which said that placing a human artifact on a hill in Tennessee changes everything about the hill and Tennessee. Consciousness places frames of meaning on the wilderness.

That's what I see in the look in Beau's eyes. It's entirely likely, as Stevens is his favorite poet. And it is a gorgeous day, with the scent of sand and pine adrift like microscopic confetti in the morning breeze, and I do enjoy walking.

Unleashed

CAROLYNNE SCOTT

I n the evening, along about nine, when the stresses of the day have subsided, I offer myself a special reward—a walk through my neighborhood.

If I don't get up and get going, Buddy, my Labrador retriever, reminds me with a nudge of his caramel-colored nose. "All right," I say, and proceed to gather my keys, my long black flashlight, and his leash.

In seconds, we are out the door and enjoying ourselves as we pass beneath my neighbor's huge chestnut tree. There are plenty of streetlights, and all the houses are well illuminated. Having been mugged by daylight somehow makes me less fearful of the nighttime which wraps us like a velvet cloak.

The leash remains in my pocket, as does my secret tear gas container which I often forget anyway. We walk up 53rd Street and stop to sniff the blooming pyracantha bushes along the periphery of the Girls' Club property and then, a moment later, pause to enjoy the splendid yellow and red roses climbing a fence at the house on the corner. In summertime, we admire the green beans growing along wire fencing at the same house, or the yellow squash blooming in a big clay pot. There's no embarrassment about ogling other people's yards in the dark.

Buddy waits for me at the corner if he has wandered ahead, but if there is anything or anybody in sight, I command him to "Stay close," and he trots back to my side. When he first adopted us, I'd use the leash, and he would weave back and forth tripping me up. Finally, in the dark, we discovered there is no need for a leash. There never is with real love.

Sometimes along 7th Court, we will see Juanita Weekly setting her garbage can out and reminisce about our days on the *Birmingham Post-Herald,* or we'll pass by the house where other Labs (with proper papers) are one-by-one training for field trials in Virginia, and Buddy will do his major sniffing. Sometimes we'll turn left at 54th and go by the white brick house where Miss Myrtle Jones Steele taught all us Crestwood kids to play the piano. Buddy stops to speak to an Australian shepherd fenced there. That same dog by day has been known to growl and snap when they're both on leashes. The cool of the evening has its balm.

One front porch we pass is populated with people who are swinging and laughing and talking. They wave to us; Buddy wags, and I say hello. It's amazing how sharp, neat and clean all the houses look in the dark. By day, we might see some peeling paint or dirty windows; by night everything sparkles.

This routine is not reserved for summer. We do it in every kind of weather, even sprinkling rain or when it's cold as ice. I feel positively cheated when there's an evening thunderstorm and Buddy has gone under the bed. I miss the outside air.

My twenty-year-old son has quit preaching to me about the dangers of my nightly peregrinations, because I always retort that we saw nobody the least bit threatening. A 120-pound dog would deter anybody. And, the exercise is vital to my blood sugar control. (I'm a Type II.)

Once when a wolf-husky and his little cream-colored accomplice decided to one-up Buddy, he stood perfectly still with his neck in the bigger dog's mouth. I gave it a loud sermon and short squirt of tear gas, and we walked away.

I find that I am more in touch with the moon since these night walks began, and the stars hold the endless fascination they did when as a child I sat with my family on the patio of another house in Crestwood and looked for the Big Dipper.

Sometimes (six blocks later) when we get back home, Buddy looks like he would like to stroll farther—perhaps to his own doggy haunts, but I cajole him toward the backyard for a quick game of toss and fetch, and finally we go in, rewarded, rejuvenated and resilient against the coming day.

The Message of the Fox

Vicki Noll

For the last six years, I have walked the same 2-mile path, a stretch of asphalt between two separate farms. Corn, wheat, and alfalfa grow in a planned rotation with a pattern that escapes me. One field sits unplowed, inhabited by wildflowers. A stand of trees on the east side of the road is balanced by thick woods to the west. At the end of the road, a huge oak creates a stark silhouette against the Ohio sky.

At one time, I paid no attention to these things. My walk was an unconscious habit like brushing my teeth, made bearable only by audio books that droned in my ears. I fixed my eyes on the road, barely noticing the scenery.

In Native-American spirituality, it's believed that nature sends soul-nurturing messages to the receptive human listener. A Huron proverb says, "Listen to the voice of nature, for it holds treasures for you." Accordingly, every animal that crosses one's path does so for a reason. Every tree, rock, and flower is a gift waiting for the right person to receive it. But as I wandered with my headphones on, lost in taped mysteries, I was not a receptive listener.

Then a skinny red fox stepped into the road just 10 feet away from me. In an instant, all my senses were focused. I didn't want to breathe, and it seemed he didn't either.

For a full minute, we eyed each other across a short distance. I took in his small form, his spindle-thin legs and alert eyes. I smelled his musty, wet-dog odor. Although he was compact, I didn't underestimate his power or my vulnerability. My fear, though, was quieted by gratitude for this rare meeting. We maintained eye contact until he blinked, then continued his trek across the road into the waist-high corn.

Whatever mystery novel blared through the earphones was lost in the mystery I had just witnessed. I continued my walk in quiet amazement, watching the fields for signs of him, wondering what message had been sent to me on the back of the fox. As I searched, I saw white-wrapped rolls of hay dotting the fields like giant marshmallows. I saw alfalfa guarded by blue wildflowers with military-straight stems. Milkweed pods in the first trimester presided over the empty field. A sole honey locust sapling stood there proudly in the midst of a meadow. I thought, had these wonders always awaited me?

Each day since, I have listened for other messages from nature. I've abandoned the audio books and look up from the pavement. I've opened my senses. Having discovered the sacred in the mundane, I await the surprises that an ordinary walk will bring. I hear nature's whispers.

You Can Go Home Again

NED STUCKEY-FRENCH

I t is the end of May, and Elizabeth and I are taking a walk along an abandoned spur of railroad tracks out of town, as we do most evenings after dinner. Here, on the Indiana prairie, we can see for miles. The sun is setting behind a wall of cumulus clouds, heaped and boiling. A front is coming in from the northwest.

As we walk, I think about what I will teach my high school juniors tomorrow. We'll start with a mini-lesson on dangling modifiers, but we'll spend most of the hour on *Huck Finn*. I'm not sure how to teach it—the students are tired of their small towns and so was Huck, but their options are different than his. There's no "Territory" left to "light out for." They will end up in big cities—Chicago or Indianapolis, if they leave at all.

Elizabeth and I grew up in Indiana, but we each lived and worked for several years out East. I was a union organizer in Boston, and Elizabeth, a social worker in Virginia Beach. Three years ago, we came home to Indiana, where we met and fell in love. On our wedding invitations we quoted *The Great Gatsby:* "So when the blue smoke of brittle leaves was in the air and the wind blew the wet laundry stiff on the line I decided to come back home."

We leave the railroad tracks and cross the fields, stepping deliberately over the little corn plants until we get to our destination—an unused silo that stands by itself like a bunker. We climb the 40-foot ladder carefully. At the top we perch ourselves where we can see forever, or at least almost to Illinois. Elizabeth repeats what one of us always says up there: "It flattens out real nice, doesn't it?" We laugh at our private joke. The breeze gusting in ahead of the front gathers force and blows our voices away, so we just sit and look. Dust devils scurry across the field. A cat hunts in the shadows along a fence row. Swallows and purple martins swoop below us, harvesting mosquitoes and gnats.

As the sun set, lights come on in the farmhouses. The closest one, maybe half a mile away, is the Gepharts' place. Sally Gephart is in my third-period journalism class. Her father farms the land between here and Little Pine Creek. I think the light I see is coming from the window above their kitchen sink. It's fluid and green, as if from an aquarium. Farther out, most of the lights are brighter and have a blue or orange tint.

My students always ask why I left Boston for Indiana. If I could move the class up here, maybe I could show them the beauty of their cornfields, their train tracks, their farm lights.

The dots of light farthest away flicker and disappear and flicker on again. I imagine they are kerosene lamps setting aglow the mica windows of sod huts, or even the cooking fires at the hunting camps of the Sioux who followed the buffalo down from the Dakotas. Thickets of underbrush and scrub oak that mark the peat bogs into which mastodons stumbled and sank disappear into the darkness. In the sky, Venus appears and then, one by one, the stars.

In a few minutes, we'll climb down from the silo and walk home. Perhaps, like Elizabeth and me, my students will have to leave before they can return.

The Dead of Winter

Suzanne Strempek Shea

In the winter, four or five mornings a week, I head to the cemetery.

Sure, I have other options in my New England village. But when snow falls, the road to the cemetery is reliably plowed. December through April, the Sts. Peter and Paul Cemetery becomes my track.

It's not a big place. Only several acres of the huge field are currently taken up by plots. But it has a loop of three connecting driveways and a long paved avenue ideal for walking.

My dog and I walk the pavement at a brisk clip, fast enough to keep Homer at a decent trot and me warm enough to ignore whatever the thermometer has sunk to. Quickly we move past the headstones, many engraved with names from my own life story. This is my parish cemetery, and the majority of those buried here once lived in my town, some on my street, several in my own home. My grandparents are buried here, as is my father. As is the girl who for 20 years was my best friend.

The names blur as Homer and I pass, as surnames on mailboxes did during my childhood bike rides: Sakowski, Pardo, Pytka, Zyblot, Wojtowicz. Moving back down the same little road, now facing the backs of the markers, I see first names and dates that framed each person's time here. Born at the end of the last century, or during the Depression, or before World War II. Or the same year that I was.

I stride past the stone for the man who never failed to buy two packages of 4-H cookies from me when I arrived with my little wagon. I pass one for a woman who played whist with my grandmother and who, I learned from her marker, had once been a nurse in the Army. And one for the man who owned Chubby, the cocker spaniel I used to walk solo on a length of clothesline and pretend was mine. There's one for a kid from my class, initials D.M., who said he wanted to be a doctor, and we all thought it was great that he'd be "D.M. the M.D." But he never got the chance. Stories flash like a circle of transparencies in my old View-Master, one click for each of the lives and those big and small things I knew about them.

I have friends who in bad weather walk their neat sidewalks or around sheltered malls and gymnasium tracks. Some descend into cellars, sentencing themselves to a certain number of minutes on ski machines or stationary bikes. Others put their routines on hold and wait for better weather.

All these people I invite to the cemetery.

Few take up the offer. Most see it as depressing.

Far from it. Walking the cemetery, I am energized by the mere fact that I am there. Looking, remembering, thinking, pacing my steps to the thoughts that silence nurtures in my mind. I think about what I'll do that day, this evening, tomorrow, and beyond. I think about how right now, this morning, it feels good simply to be alive. While it's still my turn.

Sharing the Road: Parents, Children, and Lovers

Embracing the Hour

Faith Coley Salie

We were out on a walk when we discovered my mother's cancer had returned. For a year and a half after her surgery, we had lulled ourselves into a sense of calm about her health. But that day my youthful 52-year-old mother stopped short and held her chest in pain. Seeing her like that, alternately wincing and laughing at the shock of it all, I knew something was profoundly wrong.

"Our walk," as we always called it, started when I was 17 and determined to lose weight. The route never varied, nor did the time: 3½ miles in an hour, through our Atlanta suburb, rain or shine. As the weight came off, our walk evolved. More than exercise, our hour gave me a chance to know my mother as a woman and a friend. Over the course of nine years we walked, daily while I was in high school, picking it up again when I returned home from college, or from abroad, or for the holidays.

As we walked, of course, we talked. In those hours, I learned about my mother's childhood—her summers on Cape Cod, the housekeeper who smelled of orange blossoms. About her father, who died when she was 26. About telling my grandmother she was going to be a nun, then ultimately juggling four marriage proposals. She told me about her pregnancies and even recommended a personal lubricant. Back in 1988, while rain fell on my fresh perm, Mom ran home for an umbrella as I sought shelter in a stranger's garage. And when it snowed, we bundled ourselves up to the point a neighbor once stopped and offered to drive us to whoever's house we were due to clean.

After her cancer came back, Mom underwent chemotherapy. She insisted on walking through treatments. We bought her a hat with blond hair attached to the brim. Mom got a kick out of taking it off as soon as we stepped into the house to reveal her hot, bald head. I was conscious, though, of her increasing shortness of breath. For the first time, I had to slow down for her. We never considered stopping. Too much was at stake. My mother's ability to walk gave her dignity in the face of a disease that took away her hair, her strength, and finally her life. But sometimes we slowed our pace so she could put her arm around me as I cried. We kept walking until the cancer cracked her back, one month before she died.

As I entered the church for Mom's funeral, a childhood neighbor approached me with her mother. Mom and I had regularly waved to this pair as we passed by them on our walks. They told me that after hearing of Mom's death, they decided to walk together, as they'd seen us do for a decade. They wanted to spend time together and learn more about each other.

Since my mother's death, I've stopped walking and started running instead. Walking is still too painful. I'd rather not stop to wonder about the name of a flower without my mother there to enlighten me. Someday, though, I will walk again. And on those walks, I will tell my daughter everything I can about my best friend, her grandmother.

Two for the Trail

HOLLY LOVE

'm always apprehensive about suggesting the plan for a romantic date. Am I imposing my own preferences, I wonder? Am I picking an activity that's too expensive, too intimate, or too corny? My anxiety over this was especially high at the beginning of my relationship with Sean. Better let him decide these things. After all, he had lost his sight three years before to diabetes. What he could and could not do seemed to me a delicate issue.

But then, Sean was the one to suggest renting a movie. Together we "watched" *Mr. Holland's Opus,* and he heard things in the film that I could not see. That was when I stopped underestimating his range of experience.

Sean knew that I walked three miles every day. Hesitantly, I invited him to join me in a jaunt through Pennsylvania's Ridley Creek State Park. He replied, "I thought you'd never ask."

It was November, no less. Sean didn't balk at the cold, despite his diabetes-related circulation problems. Still agile underneath four clothing layers and a pair of serious sneakers for extra foot protection (also a concern of diabetics), he faced the paved trail and let his trust in me do the walking.

The trail would be different for Sean than his familiar territory of suburbia, where on solitary strolls he always used his white cane to detect sidewalk rises, curbs, and obstacles like stop signs and trash cans. Here there would be smoother, wider ground flanked by forest and streams and traversed by runners, cyclists, and dogs. I felt intensely privileged to be his nature guide.

Finally I had a good excuse to take a smell-the-flowers ramble, instead of my usual fourteen-minutes-per-mile power walk. Sean hadn't walked fast since going blind. We started out moving slowly with our arms linked and with him still relying on his cane.

"Can you hear the waterfall coming up on the right?" I asked him. It was one of my favorite spots on the path.

"What do you think?" he answered with a smile. "I can hear it. I can also feel the cooler air."

Sean held on to my waist from behind to follow me over some tree roots closer to the cascading water, where he stole a kiss by an oak tree. I'd always suspected waterfalls were romantic, but recently I'd been drinking them in alone.

Sean then reached a comfort level that allowed him to fold up and put away his cane. "Is there a hillside to our left?" he asked further down the trail. I was amazed, because there was. He explained that he could sense when open space became less open. Likewise, on his neighborhood walks, he said he frequently put his hand out to reach for a tree that he could tell was there because of the interruption of traffic sound waves.

I suddenly felt impaired by my reliance on sight in the wilderness. I'd never before considered paying attention to the nuances he perceived. Exploring his sensual acumen was engrossing.

"So, it must smell quite different here than on the streets around your house. Better, right?" I asked.

"Yes. More natural. Fresher. But you know what smells really good? You."

"Hey," I said playfully. "We're supposed to be enjoying the setting here."

"That's all I'm doing."

Sean might have been a bit unnerved the first few times a cyclist whizzed by at close range, but he quickly adjusted. I continued directing him around klatches of park visitors for a half mile, wavering between describing the scenery and keeping my mouth shut. By telling him there was a ray of sunshine piercing a trio of beeches, would I only make him feel worse that he could no longer enjoy the sight of them? Years before he had enjoyed gazing out over mountains in Oregon. He had spent summers at the New Jersey seashore watching balmy sunshine light up lazy tides. I expressed this concern about stirring visual memories.

"Life is a richer adventure for me than you might imagine," he assured me. "I can still feel the sun, and the wind, and you on my arm. Your descriptions are icing on the cake. Please ice away." That was a relief to hear. Since we are both writers (we'd met in a writing class), it would have been hard for either one of us to keep our observations to ourselves.

"Okay, then. The thing that's just caught my eye is the barreling St. Bernard on the other side of the path." It was like "I Spy" for grown-ups, and it was always my turn. We sat down on a bench as another dog and owner brushed by us. I couldn't resist petting the dog, and Sean joined in. Even after a few minutes, we were sure the owner did not know that my companion was blind. There were a lot of people wearing sunglasses out there that day.

As we started walking again, I asked Sean, "I have to know. Do you have the urge to go faster . . . to get your heart pumping a little more? We could hold hands instead of linking arms, and you'd be absolutely safe. Do you want to try it?"

Both his desire to move freely and to impress me factored into his answer. "Yes. Let's."

We proceeded faster, fingers entwined. In a few minutes, though, he told me he was ready to let go of my hand. His confidence in me felt wondrous. Putting *more* physical distance between us actually brought us closer.

We approached a little tunnel built under a minor roadway. I'd been through it countless times before and knew that even the acoustics of one's breathing changed when underneath it. Sean noticed right away, of course. We played a few echo games in there, and I decided not to care that other people were staring.

"I think it's time for you to try walking with your eyes closed," Sean said. "See if you can stay straight."

I could only manage to take five steps before opening my eyes, and then found myself even further off the path than I'd predicted. That gave me new admiration for Sean. Every day he had to access a special sense of direction that the sighted never do. I'd started out feeling as though I were doing Sean some sort of favor by decreasing my exercise pace and distance in order to escort him. It turned out that he did me a much bigger favor, by showing me what a bouquet for the senses walking really is. Not even taste is left out, I realized—more than a few gnats and snowflakes and scarf lint particles have landed on my lips in three decades of walks.

"This was a good idea," Sean said when we made it back to the car, hugging me.

"Do you mean coming to the park today, or dating me?" I teased.

"Ah, good question," he said. "I'll tell you the answer on our next walk."

Walking for Couple Time

BETSY BANKS EPSTEIN

While raising three teenagers, my house has been a drop-in center for everybody else's children too. "How can you stand the chaos?" friends ask, fretting that I must be exhausted from the dissonance. They don't realize that by keeping company with youth, I stay young. I'm current from my clothes to my taste in music and food. How else would I know that clunky shoes are de rigueur, or that jazz is once again cutting edge? More important, how else would I get to know that new boyfriend angling to stay overnight or that girl who's willing to join us for our family vacation?

Recently a friend whose child logged many hours in our home joined me for a bowl of chili. "My son remembers you and your husband walking . . . just when the noise got really crazy . . . you'd walk," she commented and continued, "from you, he learned the importance of making time for oneself." Her observation got me thinking about those moments when just as things at home were heading out of control, my husband would look at me, grab his jacket off the hook, and plead: "We need to take a walk." As my friend pointed out as we lunched together, my husband and I have come to appreciate walking as a way to have couple time.

Over the years, we've realized that it's okay to hold hands and walk silently. Sometimes a sky glowing with hundreds of stars speaks for itself. Yet during other evenings, walking for a few miles helps us iron out mundane weekend details and decide if we're comfortable allowing two thirteen-year-olds to ride the trolley alone into the city. In an entirely different domain, walking enables us to vent our rage at a current political situation or mull over a world crisis. Walking is one of the few ways we can distance ourselves from all life's little interruptions.

Vividly I remember a balmy Saturday night when, after settling our sons in front of some videos, my husband and I laced our walking shoes for a relaxing jaunt into town and a browse at a bookstore. When we returned to our street a few hours later, we could see that all the lights in our home were blazing. Bodies were silhouetted in the living-room window; extra cars lined the driveway. Returning from a camping trip with six friends, our daughter, a junior in college, needed our house as a way station on the route back to school.

Spotting us through the doorway, she came running outside and into my arms: "Surprise! Mom!"

"I wish I had known you were coming for dinner . . . I like to cook for you . . ." I lamented.

"Don't worry, Mom, we finished the leftover Chinese food, the lasagna, and we're staying here . . . if it's okay . . . ," she replied.

My husband and I looked on while this group un-loaded their sleeping bags, and chatted about the sunny weather they'd enjoyed and the pelicans they'd photographed. We brewed espresso while they took the showers they'd yearned for. "Thanks for everything . . . I hope the commotion's no bother," one bearded fellow wondered. I felt my husband's hand on mine as we leaned back on our family-room sofa.

Sunday morning while the girls toasted bagels, the boys sliced pineapples and melons. Everyone cleared plates and scrubbed pans. As the final vehicle backed away from the curb, waves of exhaustion enveloped me.

"Let's take a walk . . . ," suggested my husband. "Even a short one will get the kinks out of our legs and the cobwebs out of our heads." As always, I relished the chance for quiet reflection with the man who has been my boyfriend for over thirty years.

City Mouse, Country Mouse

HANK HERMAN

When my first son was little, I used to take him out for a walk in his stroller most evenings. With Matt clutching a half-eaten bagel and his ever-present juice bottle, and me at the controls of his Maclaren, we'd ride down the elevator, wave to Felix (or Pete, or Van—whichever doorman was on that night), and head east to Broadway. After a stop at Mrs. Fields on 86th Street, we'd bumper-car our way down the avenue, where there was a thrill-a-block for a bright-eyed and constantly starving one-and-a-half-year-old: Herman's, the store with *our* name on it; Indian Walk, the kids' shoe store featuring a revolving bear in sneakers; Menash, the artists' bazaar that sold no-stain markers; and Häagen-Dazs, Zabar's and H&H Bagels—with *food!* At 79th Street, we'd cross Broadway, make a U-turn, and head back up the east side of the avenue to 88th—the exact same route every time.

Our stated goal was to see the moon, which was no mean feat in Manhattan: You could only manage it on select nights at certain intersections. But it didn't really matter if we spotted the moon or not; we were in it just as much for the ritual: always a chocolate chip cookie at Mrs. Fields, always touching every bar on the gate around the Church of St. Paul and St. Andrew. We were also in it for the people-watching: Upper Broadway had them all, from sleek women in leather pants walking their akitas, to street people in tattered overcoats muttering to themselves about having to erase the blackboards. And for the conversation, which consisted largely of Matt's exclaiming "I see a bus—ooooh!" He made a point of distinguishing school buses from the silver-and-blue Manhattan Transit buses: No question about it—the kid was a city mouse.

But things change. Matt grew from a toddler who liked the stroller into a boy who wanted to *run*. He was eventually joined by his kid brother, Greg. What had once seemed a spacious apartment shrank dramatically when it had to absorb two boys and their belongings. In fact, the whole city was shrinking around us: When we went out to play ball, the only playground we had was a sliver on 83rd and Riverside. Broadway was changing, too—it began to seem not so much thrilling as dirty.

We gave up the close quarters of the Upper West Side for the wide open spaces of Connecticut—and our evening stroll has changed in kind. No elevator to wait for; it's out the front door and we're off: right on Clapboard Hill, left on Turkey Hill, past the Greens Farms train station, and on down to Burying Hill Beach, to walk on the jetty and feed the swans. Instead of clutching a juice bottle, Matt throws bread crumb passes to seagulls. Here in paradise, the talk no longer revolves around buses: Greg lobbies for new Air Jordans, Matt assesses his chances of playing in the Little League All-Star game. And we can easily see the moon, spreading a corridor of light across the smooth waters of the Long Island Sound.

We don't see any people in strange outfits cursing under their breath, but we do often see deer, woodchucks, and kids on Rollerblades. And if we catch high tide, we kick off our sneakers and wade in. It's an idyllic scene—all we bargained for, and then some. We're country mice now. But something makes me nostalgic, and I don't think it's Zabar's or H&H Bagels or the bright lights of Broadway that I miss.

I think it's that little kid in the stroller.

Footsteps

Beth Mund

I have recently slid belly first into my eighth month of pregnancy. My soon-to-be son and I have walked through each trimester leaving behind, along with my favorite pair of tight-fitting jeans, many miles of traveled suburban neighborhoods. I have returned curious stares at my belly from sedentary onlookers with only a smile, knowing that the miles I clock are my safety net beneath the balancing act of hormonal instability. Calming and soothing, they are my daily epidural, numbing all sense of pain and discomfort.

As I prepare for my walk this afternoon, I sense the coldness of the January afternoon, and pull on my long underwear, maternity turtleneck, and faded blue collegiate sweatshirt. I feel like a newborn baby snugly bundled in a receiving blanket, ready to brace the outside world. I glance out the window and am surprised to see the first snowfall of the winter. Suddenly, the growing life inside of me is waking up, kicking away as if he is telling me to stop stalling, and get on my sneakers. "Okay, let's get out there!" I say, as I tie my laces, reach for my mittens, and pull on my blue checkered fleece jacket.

It is snowing harder as I begin my journey. Cottony balls of coldness drift lazily to the ground with not a care in the world. Each flake is a cleanly sculptured work of art looking like clones of one another, yet having some minuscule difference that cannot be seen by the naked eye. Walking through the fallen snow with my child to be, I have a feeling of being part of a larger designed plan affecting generations of life that have come and gone before me, and those yet to be born.

I turn the corner and feel the cold snow being thrust upon my already aching ears. I pick up my pace and feel the rhythm of my arms and legs working together to carry the weight of my protruding stomach, attempting to keep my awkward 150-pound frame upright and balanced. My mind is racing along with my body. Thoughts of baby names and lullabies swarm around in my head.

The first mile sneaks up on me. I can feel the oxygen pumping through my lungs, traveling through my blood, flowing with a purpose like a river downstream. It is seeping from my body, through my lifeline, to my child, pumping wellness and health into his growing little body. He has gone back to sleep. The rhythm of my steps has both calmed and soothed him. How very strange that the life inside of me is soothed by my constant motion, and grows alert when I am still.

The cars pass by, one by one, with windshield wipers trying to keep pace with the falling snow. After a while, I do not notice the cars, or the cold. My arms and legs continue to work carrying me to the end of my third and final mile. As I turn down Lindsey Court, I see the lights of my house, which in the grayness of the cloudy afternoon, appear brighter than normal. I notice the snow-covered driveway and turn around to see my footsteps. They are disappearing as quickly as they were made, but I know they exist. I know from the redness of my cheeks, and the sense of tranquility in my head that they carried me through my walk. I tilt my head toward my belly and whisper, "Soon you'll be following in my footsteps, but until then, I will do the walking for both of us."

Just Strolling Along

JODI RUSCH LEAS

M y daily walking program was on a roll until my son, Nicholas, decided he no longer wanted to be pushed in the stroller. He had just turned one, started walking on his own and decided buggies were for babies not for big boys.

Up until that time, I had enjoyed a vigorous workout—pushing 25 pounds of stroller and strapping infant, 45 minutes two times a day. After nine months of pregnancy, during which I watched my stomach stretch and sag like a water balloon, my daily walks helped my abdominal muscles tighten, my calf muscles strengthen, and perhaps, most important for a first-time mom, my mind relax.

Oh, how I loved my walks. Nicholas and I would head out the back door, the sun shining on our faces, the wind blowing on our backs. My son would either sit erect, his eyes aglow, pointing to everything we passed by—children dressed in blue jeans and T-shirts, playing Wiffle ball in the park; an ice-cream truck, its windows frosty white, rounding the corner near our house; the paper boy, a gray sack slung over his shoulder, tossing newspapers in front yards. Or else he would lie back, his eyes closed in half-moon shapes, cooing softly as if to say, "Mom, I love our walks too."

Our peaceful bliss came to an end the day Nicholas discovered his newfound freedom—walking. When he realized his own 15-inch legs could propel him wherever he wanted to go whenever he wanted to go, he was no longer content to sit in the stroller. I'll never forget the last time I tried to take him for a walk. We were about two miles from home, winding through the neighborhoods which surround our house, when Nicholas stood up and jumped out of the stroller.

"Get back here," I yelled. But Nicholas didn't listen. Not only had he learned to walk, he had also cultivated another skill: ignoring his mother. There was only one thing he wanted and one thing only. He wanted to walk. And walk he did. Up the nearest driveway, into a pile of dirt, behind garbage cans, over a neighbor's newly planted flower garden, and into oncoming traffic.

At that point I had had it. Nicholas didn't want to be pushed in the stroller any longer, but I didn't want to be pushed around by him either. Plus, I wasn't going to let a one-year-old get in the way of my workout. I picked him up and tossed him in the stroller, pulling the strap hard and buckling him in tight.

He kicked. He screamed. He howled like a dog locked in a kennel. Finally, my stubborn son wiggled himself free.

I grabbed him again and lifted him up, determined to get home as soon as possible even if it meant carrying him all the way back. But he wanted nothing to do with it, his mouth pouting, his legs thrashing, his arms pounding against my chest.

"You are a naughty boy," I said. "I can't believe what a bad boy mommy has."

Embarrassed by this public outburst, both his and mine, I looked around to see if anyone was watching. The streets were empty; I didn't see anyone else around. But as Nicholas and I continued our struggle down the sidewalk, I saw someone approaching us. It was another mother taking her son for a walk. He was about eight years old. The mother stood behind her son pushing him not in a stroller but in a wheelchair. He sat perfectly still. He wasn't able to crawl out of the wheelchair. He wasn't able to move his legs at all.

At that moment, I squeezed my son and felt his tiny, yet powerful legs pushing against my stomach. And I realized how lucky I was to have a son who could jump out of his stroller, who could walk away from me, who could ignore my pleas to sit still.

I put my son back down on the sidewalk, pushing the stroller in one hand and in the other holding my son's small hand. And he was fine. That was all he wanted—to walk side by side with me. It seemed silly to have gotten so upset because my son didn't want to sit in his stroller.

After all, he and I were no different; we both wanted the same thing. To simply go for a walk on our own two feet. To feel our legs moving. Our hearts beating. Our minds stretching. Our souls relaxing. To feel gloriously alive as we walked hand in hand together. Soon the stroller would find its way to the attic next to the bottles, beside the bassinet. But as I pushed it down the street for the last time, its wheel spinning round, I realized the important lesson the stroller taught me: how I needed to learn to roll with the changes in my son's life.

The World According to Allie

BILL DONAHUE

For most of July, the boundary was the edge of the yard. Allie, my 13-month-old daughter, could play in the grass and in the trickle of hose water that we sometimes ran on the marigolds. But if she toddled past the driveway, we grabbed her, and she'd arch her back, screaming. She'd watched both of us, her mother and me, venture past the corner— she'd seen us disappear like ships off the edge of the world, and now she wanted to know what was Out There.

Our city block is on a fairly steep hill. Earthquakes and frost heaves have ripped cracks in the pavement, and skateboarders slalom amid the pedestrians—it was not a place for a baby. But one night Allie elbowed me in the ribs hard. We were going.

Down Alder Street first—past the Dalmatian who churns inside his fence, past the vegetable patch on the corner and—what was this?—on toward a telephone pole with a long wire anchoring it to the ground. Allie batted the wire so it sang like a guitar, then scrambled back toward the vegetables to pick at the lettuce. I'd seen this routine before, of course. As a parent, you get used to the sputtering chaos, and you try, as best you can, to go forward: Get out of the store before your kid sees the candy. Get out of the lettuce before your neighbor shows up with an admonishing scowl. I reached for Allie, but she wobbled past me, her tiny legs jerking like a new marionette. She stepped onto the pavement, then crashed. There was blood on her knee.

She shrieked; I held her. I patted the soft blonde down on her head, but still she sobbed on, twisting and raucously kicking until, finally, I just set her down. I had to.

Now there were baby carriages on the street and cats who'd come out in the cool of the evening to slink through the grass. Allie chased after a marmalade kitten, then stumbled upon two plastic flamingos, which, valiantly, she tried to pry free.

It was absurd. Usually, it took me less than 3 minutes to reach these flamingos; Allie and I had been out for nearly an hour. All that kept me going was this: Somehow, miraculously, we were making our way around the block. We were closing in on the third corner. My kid was going to pull this one off.

We kept going—past the house with the mossy rocks in the yard, then over a metal grate that clanged wonderfully when you leapt on it. At the last corner, there were pinecones. Allie grabbed one; squealing, she pushed it up toward my hip. I laughed, but then she flailed her arms at me, grunting. No words (she couldn't talk then), but still she made me remember a hike I took once on a trail that cut through a rock tunnel under a waterfall: I stood inside the tunnel and felt the rock shake. That surprised me, and now Allie was just as surprised by this pinecone. It was new to her, and she was scraping it on my leg. "Wake up, Pop," she was trying to tell me. "The world is a luminous thing."

I took that bristly cone—and the next one, and the next one, until my arms filled and I started using my pockets. But then Allie spun off, and I had to drop the cones on the sidewalk. We went home (yes, all the way around the block), and Allie climbed into her crib. Like a wild animal after a feast, she fell quickly asleep.

Around the Kitchen and Across Vermont

TOM GLICK

I was fascinated by states as a kid. I knew every fact, figure, curve, and angle of each of them. I even slept with my United States of America puzzle pieces. The panhandle of Texas jabbed my side when I turned over at night, and California was sticky with spilled orange juice and doughnut goo.

My fascination with the states drove my mother crazy. At first she thought she had a smart little boy. But when I started walking around the house for hours pretending to cross all the states in our white 1980 Volvo, she realized she had a crazy little boy. I spent enough time in the backseat of our car while my parents ran weekly errands to the grocery store, that I knew I wanted to travel on my own terms. The least I could do was make car noises in the living room. I said, "Vvvroooom, how many hours does it take to get through New York, Mom?"

"Oh, about four, I guess."

I walked around the house for four hours.

"Mom, the northwest tip of Pennsylvania is next. How many hours?"

"Forty-five minutes maybe."

Forty-five minutes later: "And Ohio, how many hours, Mom?"

My mother was too honest. She should have told me fifteen minutes, or at least told me to sit down and pretend to travel. But she always told me the truth, and I spent a large percentage of my childhood walking in circles because of it.

One evening when I was driving through New York, I heard my mom ask my dad, "Couldn't you tell him to do that somewhere else? He's wearing out my carpet."

I heard my father say—and I remember it well; it was a prophecy to last a lifetime—"That boy has a mind of his own."

While I walked, I tried to precipitate adulthood by partaking in another seemingly inane activity. Even though I didn't know how to read yet, I carried a book with me, sometimes two, turning the pages and scanning the words as I swerved around my mother and the toys I left on the floor, pretending to read like any adult might on a long road trip.

One of the first books I ever picked up was Peter Jenkins's *The Walk West*, a sequel to *A Walk Across America*. I understood the title and was instantly enthralled. When I carried it with me on my adventures around the house, I felt like I was really going somewhere, not in circles around our kitchen, but across enough actual terrain to make my feet ache—a sacrifice I thought would make my hero, Peter Jenkins, proud.

Another hero of mine, a Peter Jenkins admirer himself, encouraged my wandering feet (and mind) at an early age. Conveniently, I didn't have to know how to read to be influenced by him. This second hero was my dad. He knew the minute I could name all fifty states in fifty seconds that I would go somewhere in life, not just around in circles. He condoned my walking fantasies and suggested one weekend that we walk across our home state of Vermont.

My mother was leery. I was only ten. But Vermont is a small state, so she thought I might be able to handle it. One Saturday morning at 4:00 A.M., my mother and brother drove my dad and me the width of Vermont to where we would start walking back the sixty miles to get home. I thought it was Christmas. We were really going to walk for hours, and get somewhere!

I made sure that we crossed the line into New York before the walk began. We were going to cover every square inch of all 59.9 Vermont-wide miles. The exercise would be for naught if we missed even one. Seeing the "Welcome to Vermont" sign was particularly exciting for me. As we walked past it that foggy morning, inaugurating our long trek to New Hampshire, I yelled, "BOOP!" to signal that we had started our trip.

Truth be known, I had not yet developed the physical prowess it takes to walk across even a tiny state like Vermont. On the second day, as we ascended Killington Mountain in the pouring rain, I would sooner have taken steps to transform myself into a garden vegetable than take steps toward the New Hampshire border. I was drenched and sore from the day before, and the mountain kept rising in steeper grades until we were in the clouds, face-to-face with the agents that rendered me miserable.

I had a fever by the afternoon and we were still walking in the rain. We walked twenty miles for two days in a row, wet the whole way. Dad, a doctor, fed me children's Tylenol like it was candy. If only Mother knew. What kind of father would walk with his sick son on the side of the road in the pelting rain all day with only the promise of more walking the next day? Not a father who is upholding the ethics of the Hippocratic oath, I would say. Or does a father's understanding of his son transcend the ethics of medicine? Perhaps he simply realized that ten-year-olds know more about where they are going than most adults give them credit for.

A discovery that I made during the second day of the walk, to which almost every adult will attest and accept as truth, even from the squeaky pre-pubescent voice of a child, is that caffeine is wonderful. The walk across Vermont was the first time I realized its wonders. That afternoon, as we descended the other side of Killington—the mountain obstacle that had accentuated the pain of my juicy morning blisters—I almost quit. Painfully, I realized that walking downhill only chafed my blisters from different angles. Dad noticed I was dragging, so he said, "Tom, you need some caffeine."

What a doctor. What a dad! He knew best. Coffee was so much more effective than children's Tylenol. Adult juice, I called it then. It perked me up on that second day when all I wanted to do was ride home in the backseat of our Volvo.

By the end of the third twenty-mile day, as we crossed the Connecticut River into New Hampshire, my mother and brother were there to pick us up. I had such a fever (it was 103) that I couldn't even recognize my own feat. I don't remember the party my family had planned for me. I do remember being so pooped that I was immediately sent to bed while my mom and dad undoubtedly debated the fundamentals and responsibilities of parenting.

I don't know if I'll share such crazy adventures with my kids. If I do, I'll have to consult my dad to determine the dosage of Tylenol to give to them when they're soaked to the bone on the side of the road. He always seemed to know just what kind of medicine I needed. If I can give my son or daughter the same encouragement and spirit of adventure that he bestowed upon me, their ten-year-old aspirations may far exceed a three-day trek across Vermont. Whether it's around the world or around the kitchen, I'll walk with them.

Spare the Walk . . .

KATHRYN DAWSON

My parents spanked me only once when I was growing up. I don't remember what crime I'd committed, but it must have been pretty bad, because our normal discipline wasn't corporal punishment or even being deprived of certain key privileges: It was a walk around the block.

With four kids in a tiny two-bedroom house in Tucson, Ariz., the conditions were perfect for us to bicker—and we did. When the squabbling reached a certain decibel level, my father would point to the door: "All right guys, around the block." Reluctant and lingering, we would go outside, protesting, "How come none of our friends have to do this?"

I'd begin the walk with the indignant stride of a martyr, my siblings matching my steps in a similar huff. We'll get this ridiculous punishment over with, and then we'll never speak to our parents again. There was an unspoken pact: we would not, could not at any time actually enjoy the walk. The plan was to build on our initial resentment so much that when we returned home we'd be in even fouler moods than before. They'll suffer the consequences of being so unfair. They'll rue the day they inflicted such torture upon us.

Yet despite our best efforts to keep the mood hostile, we couldn't help but notice the things outside the circle of our wrath. The huge anthill with its trail of toiling workers had grown since our previous walk. The spooky lady's house came next, and we'd experience a delicious, palpable moment of terror as we passed her porch. Horned lizards, tortoises, toads, and other desert wildlife would invariably cross our path and divert our anger. By the time we reached our porch, our anger had somehow dissipated. Sometimes we even forgot to suppress any visible signs of enjoyment before opening the door.

Perhaps my parents were ahead of their time, knowing that a walk was restorative, that it could give us time to reflect upon the bigger picture and exercise our bodies. Or maybe they just wanted to enjoy the peace of a quiet home. On rare occasions we would complete our walk and immediately pick up whining from where we'd left off. My father had no compunction about repeating the punishment, so around the block we'd go again. But more often, we came back forgetting who had done what injustice to whom. Serenity reigned—until the next crisis arose. Since we were normal kids and our house didn't grow any bigger, we walked around the block on a regular basis. We came to know that neighborhood quite intimately.

At the age of 40, I've long since admitted to my parents how much I appreciated their "Spare the walk and spoil the child" creed. While my friends were being grounded or spanked, I "had" to walk. I griped about it then, but from those walks I developed a love of the outdoors, a healthy method for working out frustrations, and some dynamite calf muscles. Since then, I've worn out many pairs of sneakers taking my problems around the block. And if, when I return home, I still don't have them solved, at least I may have found an anthill or two.

Walkers and the Rest of the World

Exhilarations of the Road

JOHN BURROUGHS

O ccasionally on the sidewalk, amid the dapper, swiftly moving, high-heeled boots and gaiters, I catch a glimpse of the naked human foot. Nimbly it scuffs along, the toes spread, the sides flatten, the heel protrudes; it grasps the curbing, or bends to the form of the uneven surfaces—a thing sensuous and alive, that seems to take cognizance of whatever it touches or passes. How primitive and uncivil it looks in such company—a real barbarian in the parlour! We are so unused to the human anatomy, to simple, unadorned nature, that it looks a little repulsive; but it is beautiful for all that . . . It is the symbol of my order, the Order of Walkers. . . .

When I see the discomforts that able-bodied American men will put up with rather than go a mile or half a mile on foot, the abuses they will tolerate and encourage, crowding the streetcar on a little fall in the temperature or the appearance of an inch or two of snow, packing up to overflowing, dangling to the straps, treading on each other's toes, breathing each other's breaths, crushing the women and children, hanging by tooth and nail to a square inch of the platform, imperilling their limbs and killing the horses—I think the commonest tramp in the street has good reason to felicitate himself on his rare privilege of going afoot. Indeed, a race that neglects or despises this primitive gift, that fears the touch of the soil, that has no footpaths, no community of ownership in the land which they imply, that warns off the walker as a trespasser, that knows no way but the highway, the carriage-way, that forgets the stile, the foot-bridge, that even ignores the rights of the pedestrian in the public road, providing no escape for him but in the ditch or up the bank; that race is in a fair way to far more serious degeneracy. . . .

The human body is a steed that goes freest and longest under a light rider, and the lightest of all riders is a cheerful heart. Your sad, or morose, or embittered, or preoccupied heart settles heavily into the saddle, and the poor beast, the body, breaks down the first mile. Indeed, the heaviest thing in the world is a heavy heart. Next to that, the most burdensome to the walker is a heart not in perfect sympathy and accord with the body—a reluctant or unwilling heart. The horse and rider must not only both be willing to go the same way, but the rider must lead the way and infuse his own lightness and eagerness into the steed. Herein is no doubt our trouble, and one reason of the decay of the noble art in this country. We are unwilling walkers. We are not innocent and simple-hearted enough to enjoy a walk. We have fallen from that state of grace which capacity to enjoy a walk implies. It cannot be said that as a people we are so positively sad, or morose, or melancholic as that we are vacant of that sportiveness and surplusage of animal spirits that characterised our ancestors, and that springs from a full and harmonious life—a sound heart in accord with a sound body. A man must invest himself near at hand and in common things, and be content with a steady and moderate return, if he would know the blessedness of a cheerful heart and the sweetness of a walk over the round earth. This is a lesson the American has yet to learn—capability of amusement on a low key. He expects rapid and extraordinary returns. He would make the very elemental laws pay usury. He has nothing to invest in a walk; it is too slow, too cheap. We crave the astonishing, the exciting, the far away, and do not know the highways of the gods when we see them—always a sign of the decay of the faith and simplicity of man.

If I say to my neighbour, "Come with me, I have great wonders to show you," he pricks up his ears and comes forthwith; but when I take him on the hills under the full blaze of the sun, or along the country road, our footsteps lighted by the moon and stars, and say to him, "Behold, these are the wonders, these are the circuits of the gods, this we now tread is a morning star," he feels defrauded, and as if I had played him a trick. And yet nothing less than dilatation and enthusiasm like this is the badge of the master walker.

Walking to the Mall

BILL HARLEY

All I needed was a pair of socks. Looking out my hotel window, I could see across the highway a mall floating in the distance. Surely, there was a pair of socks at the mall. All I had to do was walk over to the mall, find a store, and buy a pair of socks. I should've suspected the metaphysical complications of walking to a mall when I tried to get some information from the hotel clerk.

"How do you get to that mall over there?" I said, "Just go over the overpass?"

"It's just two minutes," he answered. "They have 189 stores. Do you have your own car?"

"No."

"Fine, I'll call you a cab."

"Wait a minute," I said. "How do you walk over there?"

The clerk looked at me. "You want to *walk?*"

"Yeah. How far is it? A quarter, half a mile?"

"I don't know," he answered.

All the enthusiasm and color were draining from his face. He took a step away from the counter like he didn't want to be in the room with me.

"Are you sure you want to walk?"

I didn't bother to ask him directions. I could see the mall outside the window. I walked along the side of the road. There was no sidewalk. There is nothing like a sidewalk within five miles of any mall. Look for yourself. I walked along the shoulder, balancing like a tightrope walker between the rush-hour traffic on one side and a steep embankment on the other that held piles of trash.

My first major obstacle was trying to cross the ramp from the interstate to get to the overpass. When cars weren't pouring off it, they were pouring on it. The light changed and there was never a chance for me to run across. There was no walk sign. I was not supposed to be there. I became even more aware of my vulnerability, my precarious position, as I stood there waiting for a chance to dart between the cars.

As the cars went by me, they slowed to look at me. "What was that guy doing there?" Passengers had a quizzical look on their faces. I felt exposed. The whole world was passing before me and they were all thinking, "Why isn't he in a car? It must've broken down. Maybe he's a mass murderer. What is he doing out there?"

I was in the twilight zone. My deviance was obvious. I tried to appear nonchalant. I darted across the ramp and onto the bridge. There was no sidewalk on the bridge, only a one-foot lip of concrete between me and the railing and the cars screaming underneath. Cars screamed by on the other side, too, 18 inches from my path. I was not supposed to be walking to the mall. I balanced on the small path and moved along the bridge. I tried not to attract attention. I guess I did.

As I leapt off the bridge and headed toward the next exit ramp, a police car coming toward me pulled over in front of me. He leaned over and motioned for me to open the passenger door. I'm not kidding, this happened. I opened the door.

"Got a problem, buddy?" The policeman was friendly.

"No, I'm just walking to the mall."

"Did your car break down?"

"No, I was just over at the hotel over there and I thought I'd walk to the mall."

I saw the confused look on his face. He looked at the hotel then back over his shoulder to the mall.

"It's not that far," I offered in my defense.

"You want a ride?"

"No, thanks."

At the next ramp I began to feel like a homeless person, standing there waiting for something to happen to me. I looked homeless, I felt homeless. Who else but a homeless or carless person would walk to the mall?

The parking lot was in sight. There was a deep, grassy culvert I had to cross. Down at the bottom, a mysteriously green-colored liquid oozed through the grass into the pipes. The grass was tall and lush. It must be the reconstituted wetlands they built when they filled in the old ones to build the mall. I tried to leap across the marsh but didn't make it. Now I really needed new socks.

I finally reached the parking lot. It was huge. The mall seemed no closer than it had from the hotel window. I began to suspect I was chasing a mirage. I wandered across the empty spaces, thousands of them, spaces built so they could be used for two days a year. I was arriving from another planet, another dimension—the creature that walked to the mall.

I arrived at the buildings. I was on the backside of the mall. It was huge and white. It had no apparent entrance. The main entrance was a mile and a half away. I ran my hand along the stucco looking for a seam. I stumbled along the wall. A soundtrack with a 12-tone pattern with no center. I wished that I had a cart to push. I came to a door. I pushed it open, found myself standing in a storeroom. I wandered through it and finally came out on the floor.

I stood speechless, disoriented. I was standing before the women's lingerie in a major department store. A clerk seemed surprised to see me.

"My goodness. Where did you come from?"

"I walked."

"I'm sorry."

I stared at her. "I walked. I walked to the mall. Do you have any socks?" My appearance must have disturbed her. She took a step back.

She backed away out of sight and reappeared holding two pairs of socks; one was bright red, one was white.

"Which color?"

"Both."

"Great."

"How much?"

"Four-fifty each."

I stuffed $10 into her hand and grabbed the socks.

"Don't you want a bag?"

I looked at her closely. "I walked to the mall," I said. "I don't need a bag." I turned and slipped out the back door, scurried across the parking lot, waded through the marsh, weaving between cars, dancing over the bridge. I knew people were staring at me as I clutched one pair of socks in each hand. I made it to the hotel and flung the door open. The clerk looked up.

"Did you get what you needed?"

I held up the socks. "Aren't they nice?" I asked.

"Sure. Is there anything else you need?"

"Yes," I said, and leaned over the counter. "Where's a good seafood restaurant?"

"There's a great one across the street."

"Fine," I said, "make me a reservation for six o'clock."

"Fine, sir."

"And one more thing," I said as I leaned closer to him, breathing heavily.

"Yes, sir?"

"Call me a cab."

Ready, Aim, Walk

JACQUELINE TRESL

During today's walk, I was only shot at twice. Not too bad considering this is the middle of deer season. Yesterday was really awful. I ran past one field where 13 pickup trucks were parked. I heard men shouting and then—bang, bang, bang. The hunters don't actually point their guns at me and yell, "ready, aim, fire." It just feels that way. But I won't stop. Where I walk, there should be no shooting.

For 11 months out of the year, this is a you-could-hear-a-pin-drop place to walk. I cover a 6-mile loop that wanders over deer-dotted hills, turkey-laden fields, and heron-filled wetlands. If one car passes me during my 95-minute walk, it's an event.

Until November—deer season. Then, everything changes. The hordes of men from Akron and Cleveland wake in the night and drive hours to get here before dawn. Dressed in camouflage coveralls, high-powered rifles hung on their shoulders, they come for blood.

But not exactly for sport. The reason I am such an irritant to these men—and they are such a threat to me—is because of the way they hunt. A posse of men starts on the back side of a field and flushes out deer to the men waiting on the roadside. As the deer dash across the road, the men shoot. It is against the law to shoot across a road. Here, it happens every day.

So though I walk on the road, I crimp their hunting style. The first few years I walked my loop, I was stopped dozens of times by packs of hunters who advised me, "for my own good," not to walk during deer season. There I'd stand, shivering with my walker's sweat and woman-alone fear, listening to nine unwashed guys with guns telling me to get out or watch out.

Three years ago, two men appeared out of nowhere and stopped me. One of them had a long butcher knife. "Little lady," he said, "we've told you it's not safe to be out here. We might just miss the deer and you'd be our next target," moving his knife around so the sunlight glinted off the blade into my eyes.

I didn't say a word. I ran. I shaved seven minutes off my time that day. After that, I agreed to go with my husband to a gun store to look at small pistols for self-defense. The whole week, I suffered horrible nightmares about shooting people and getting sentenced to life without parole. I couldn't carry a gun.

I did agree to carry red pepper spray. Then one day I walked into a menacing dog. For once, I didn't run: I pulled the pepper spray out of my pocket and aimed. A pitiful bit of spray dripped out. The tip had clogged with lint from having been in my pocket so long. It made the dog madder. He lunged at me. I took off.

I was left with a choice. I could sit out 30 days a year, or I could defy the hunters, challenging them to go where they belong. I doubt they'll ever shoot me. None of them wants to go to jail. They just don't want anyone in their killing fields, spoiling their fun.

But I'm not in the fields, I'm on the road. And on the road I'll stay. Knives and guns and packs of mean men—as long as my legs will take me, I'll walk every day.

Auto Biography

Jim Merritt

Four years ago, for better or worse, and to the dismay of my parents and friends, I got a divorce from my car. We'd been going together since I was a teenager, but after 14 years of bad brakes, overheating, and blown gaskets, the relationship just ran out of gas.

My friends told me that I was insane, that being single, carless, and middle class in America was a social disgrace, and that by the time Friday night rolled around, with nowhere to go, I'd run crying to the nearest Hyundai dealer.

My parents scoffed, too.

"When you get stranded, don't come running home to borrow the car," my dad warned.

My mother wanted to introduce me to the daughter of an old friend who was selling a Toyota. "You're not thinking of buying a motorcycle, are you?" she asked nervously when I declined the offer.

Actually, I had something even more radical in mind: walking.

I admit, at first I missed my ex. In the morning I'd wake up and reach for my car keys, and they'd be gone. There was an empty space in the driveway where her headlights used to be. I missed her body. But soon I was ready to lace up my high-tops and get back into circulation.

It did require a little change in lifestyle. No more road trips to far-flung barbers, movie theaters, or supermarkets. I let my legs do the shopping. On the first Tuesday in November, I voted with my feet.

There were immediate compensations for my car-free existence. I stopped waking up in the middle of the night wondering if I'd left my headlights on. I threw out my jumper cables. And I swore off shock radio.

I eliminated insurance and repair bills, and used the money to do some serious traveling. (I still had to make car loan payments for my abandoned Chevy, which I considered a kind of alimony.)

When I went out on the town, I could indulge as much as I wanted without worrying about the dreaded D words, *drunk driving*. (There's no law against walking while intoxicated, as far as I know.)

And on one of the best days of my life, I took a two-hour walk along a country lane not far from my neighborhood (a 10-minute trip by car). Along the way I smelled the sea and the azaleas, picked strawberries, heard a bird cry (it proved to be an osprey), and stopped to admire a sun-drenched field straight out of van Gogh.

To be honest, I haven't stopped looking at cars. I still admire the elegance of a Mercedes and the shape of a Porsche. I've even flirted with the idea of picking up one of those new Asian models.

But after four years, I'm still a leg man, a confirmed street strider. And don't be fooled if you hear that I was cruising around town one weekend in a brand-new Buick. Contrary to rumor, it was just a rental.

Walking While You Work

JEFFREY R. KATZ

'␣ve always loved the scene in old films when the covert operative signals for his visitor to keep quiet while tilting his head toward an inanimate object in the room. He then innocently suggests the two go for a walk. Donning trench coats, they go out to plot, safely removed from microphones or eaves-droppers. I once thought only spies did business while walking. I've since discovered the walking meeting.

The first time I was caught by surprise. A few days into my first job out of college, my fiftysomething, fit-but-not-trim boss asked if I'd like to take a walk. I thought "Hey, this is easy face time. Sure, I'll take a stroll with the boss."

Eighteen floors down and two blocks away from the office, I realized I was an unprepared subordinate in the midst of a fast-paced meeting. My boss discussed the day's activities and assigned tasks while moving at a nice clip. Panicked, I searched my pockets for paper and a pen. Nothing. As we weaved through pedestrians and dodged traffic in the summer heat, my boss rapidly ticked off action items, confident that I would be the one taking action. When we reached his destination, I shot back to my desk hoping to remember half the things he said. Within a week, we were out again. This time I was prepared. With notebook and pen, I bounded after him into the elevator. The pace was frenzied, but I busily took notes (and patted myself on the back). Later, though, I was horrified to find that I couldn't read my writing.

Twice defeated, I buried my shame, and with practice, I improved. As the meetings grew more productive, their frequency increased. For my boss, the walks were an opportunity to work away from the ringing phones at our 70-person firm. For my part, I valued the time alone with my boss and the exercise. It was worth the sweat and wrinkled shirts, though my feet ached for sneakers instead of wingtips.

When I left after a year to join the Foreign Service, I was sad to say goodbye to walking meetings. Fellow diplomats overseas were not as receptive, particularly in the tropical heat of Kuala Lumpur, Malaysia. But six years later, I joined a start-up firm in New Haven, Conn. Minutes into the new job, a co-worker suggested a walk. The walking meeting was back.

Walking meetings became a staple of our new company. They allowed us to get away and focus on the big picture. Walking interviews helped screen out candidates who wouldn't thrive in our quirky culture. And we had a built-in corporate fitness program.

We walked for miles at a time, through old neighborhoods with picturesque architecture and along rivers and trails in East Rock Park. We passed children coming out to play. We felt the warmth of the summer sun, saw leaves change colors in fall, and admired frost on the trees in winter. Our creative juices flowed. Walking exercised our bodies and our minds. It drove our business.

No longer is it only John le Carré characters conducting business in parks. The walking meeting is part of the enlightened businessperson's day. But I have to get back to work—I'm going for a walk.

Learning to Walk

Judith Kirkwood

My father snaps his fingers in an army rhythm of left-right-left-right as he walks briskly down the crumbling asphalt road from our house to the new shopping center where his store is. It is 1959. He doesn't appear to make any accommodation for my shorter legs or natural inclination to dawdle, just looks back with an encouraging smile. That—and the change jingling in his pockets—is enough to help me keep up even though I have to walk double time. If I get a side ache, I think about the money I'll make cleaning the counters and straightening supplies at his popcorn shop. Usually he gives me whatever he has in his pockets that day.

The summer I am able to match him stride for stride—at about 14—my hair streams out behind me and it feels like I am flying. That is also the summer I begin working part-time with him in the store and find out what it's like to stand on a concrete floor all day, stirring caramel in a big copper kettle when it's 90 degrees outside and 110 inside. Our building is not wired for air conditioning and the sweat pours off of me, my newly acquired mask of makeup slithering down my face within minutes of my arrival.

The last thing I want to do after my shift is walk home as limp as a rag doll. But I get into the rhythm. Left, right, left, right. I can hear it in my head as I speed home to shower off the cotton candy strands that mat my hair and the caramel smell in my pores before my date picks me up. (My dad always smells like caramel.)

Born before two-car families were the norm, walking was a fact of life for me, something my car culture children cannot imagine, even though I've tried to give them some incentives from my experience.

Walking to and from school was an extended play time with friends (although we didn't have to carry 30-pound backpacks like my middle schooler does). We walked to the shopping center with friends every Saturday, so we didn't have to worry about who would pick us up and when (but the streets surrounding our mall are too busy even for adults to cross). I could take the bus, but I loved walking downtown, passing through neighborhoods of old homes with wide porches, stopping by the church for a cool drink of water, and going past the statues on the steps of the library. (Of course, we live in a subdevelopment way too far from downtown to consider walking there.)

OK. It is a different world. For one thing, I haven't done a lot of walking myself since I discovered how fast four wheels and a horn can get me to where I want to go. For another, one son is already grown up with a child of his own. But we still have options for walking together:

Walk the videos back to our neighborhood strip mall before they're overdue.

Walk to nearby restaurants to sit down and eat instead of picking up carry-out or having it delivered.

Walk our dogs to the park (in fact, there's a dog walking group in our neighborhood that includes children and adults).

Walk to the library.

Walk to the nature conservancy only a mile away to check out the prairie.

I confess, I'll never walk in a marathon or up a mountain—and my children probably won't either. But I cherish the example that my father set for me as he walked through the world. He could have gone a lot faster without me. But I think he liked the company. And so did I.

Left-right, left-right. Snap, snap, snap snap. I turn to smile at my son, who has stopped to tuck a blanket around his daughter in the stroller. He doesn't know it yet, but taking a walk with her will become one of the pure pleasures of life. And she will love him for it. I imagine my dad walking beside me always.

Walking

PAUL LINGEL

One day my car broke down and I had to walk home from work, seven miles. When I woke up the next day I walked to work, seven miles. And then I walked back home again seven miles. I did not have the opportunity to have my car repaired or buy a new car and so I continued walking to and from work each day for a total of fourteen miles a day, six days a week. I never missed a day of work, and I was never late for work (I was never late getting home either) despite whatever God, Mother Nature, or mankind threw at me in terms of weather, fatigue, or even gunshots. I walked through everything: blizzards, torrential rain, hailstorms, scorching hot heat and humidity, and subfreezing temperatures of twenty below zero.

Unlike exercise walkers, I did not have the luxury of picking and choosing which days I felt like walking or when to begin my walk, because my walk was my commute to work, and so I had to leave when I had to leave, regardless of the weather. In other words, I couldn't wait for the roads to be plowed, or the rain to stop before I began my walk, because I didn't want to be late for work. In fact, when I started walking it was the middle of January (my first day walking was the worst blizzard of the year) and I only had one pair of dress shoes to my name and no rain gear whatsoever. Not even an umbrella. I also did not have the luxury of going to a sporting goods store and buying five hundred dollars' worth of equipment before I started walking fourteen miles a day. My car broke down suddenly and unexpectedly and up to that very moment I had no idea in the world that I would find myself having to walk fourteen miles a day.

And because my walk was so long, it became the focus of my entire life. Everything I did or ate revolved around surviving the walk. In short order I learned everything that there is to know about walking by doing it far more successfully than anyone I have ever heard of or read about. Period.

During the four years and nine months that I walked fourteen miles a day, six days a week, I never took a vacation and I never got sick and I never needed medical attention. In fact, I only remember sneezing once or twice after I walked through an unbelievably nasty, freezing cold hailstorm when I had drastically underdressed. Weather reports—as you may notice—are almost totally unreliable.

After two years of walking, I was determined to walk for the rest of my life. I was sick and tired of cars breaking down and having to repair them so I did not have my driver's license renewed. Besides, I was never able to save money when I had a car. Even as a single man with two full-time jobs, and no debts, money just vaporized. As a walker, I only passed two places that were open—a bank and a supermarket.

So I would deposit my check and buy food and go home. I managed to save thousands of dollars not having a car. Before walking, I might look under my car seats for extra change!

I was not in any great physical shape before I started walking. I have size fourteen feet and they are totally flat. In fact, had I ever enlisted for military service I would have been disqualified because flat feet supposedly make you tire quickly. And I started walking when I was thirty-five years old.

I saved a life one time. I came across a young man lying in the grass, unconscious, in total darkness along the border of a state park. It was February and bitter cold. He was scantily dressed. Out of the corner of my eye I saw two police officers stop a car on a nearby highway. I hopped a few fences and told them about the emergency. The officers roused the young man and I continued my walk. If I had not found him, he would have died of hypothermia.

After four years and nine months of walking fourteen miles a day, six days a week, I applied for my driver's license again and passed the written test and the road test and they gave me a driver's license. I took my first vacation in seventeen years. I rented a car and drove along the roads that I walked. Seven miles one way looked much farther from the vantage point of a car than it did on foot. And then I drove to a motel and bought a pizza and sat down. And I thought long and hard about my journey.

Walking Victories Great and Small

Freedom Trails

KATHRYN WILKENS

The stalwart pioneer woman of stone looks as if she could stride right off her pedestal. Every day I admire her as I start my 6-mile walk along the median of a tree-lined boulevard. The statue, called "The Madonna of the Trail," honors women of the westward migration, many of whom trekked a thousand miles alongside covered wagons with their families.

Today I free my imagination and join the pioneer woman on her journey. Her work-worn hand feels rough in mine as I help her down from the pedestal. We are unusual walking companions—she in her voluminous dress, leather boots, and sunbonnet, I in shorts and a T-shirt, running shoes, and sunglasses. I tell her not to fear vehicles speeding by on either side of us as she looks askance at my bare arms and legs.

I explain to her that I walk up and down this street simply for exercise. Although I could drive a car, I walk because I want to. Afterward, I return to a home with running water and luxurious beds, a home that is warm in winter and cool in summer. I wish I had time to tell her of refrigerators, movies, and computers. I am glad there's no time to discuss nuclear war, toxic waste, and cancer.

She tells me about leaving home after packing a covered wagon with bedding, lanterns, rifles, clothing, and a plow. She complains of broken axles, lost horses, snakebite, cholera, and death. Perhaps she withholds things from me, too—the wrenching pain of leaving her parents behind to follow a husband's dream, the terror she felt when she first heard coyotes howling at dawn, or the tears she shed on her firstborn's trailside grave.

For a while, we stroll silently in the dappled shade of pepper trees and gaze up at blue-gray foothills. It dawns on us that, as different as our lives are, we are alike in one way. Our common ground is, in fact, common ground. We walk at the same speed with long, confident strides. With each step, a tiny portion of the earth's surface passes behind us. We see an ever-changing perspective. Nearer objects pass quickly. Distant objects slowly grow closer.

I realize we are restless creatures on different journeys. Hers is literal; she walks into unknown territory, seeking a place where she will begin a new life. Mine is symbolic, but I, too, am seeking something: a life enhanced by a stronger, healthier body and a clearer vision.

At the end of our walk, I look away for a moment, and when I look back, the pioneer woman is again on the pedestal. With her baby cradled in one arm, her son and rifle at her side, she strides forward forever. I see now that she is a monument not only to pioneer womanhood, but to walking itself—the very essence of freedom.

Walking Home

Brenda Williams

I t wasn't until I quit running that I finally learned
how to walk. I have always been in a hurry, strug-
gling to get places faster than anyone else, impa-
tiently swerving through the traffic of my life, hoping to arrive a few seconds earlier than the next
person. Until recent years, I had not learned the pro-
cess of life because I had been too focused on the
goals. I had time only for beginnings and endings,
not for the vacuous in-between that inhabits most of
our lives. Even if I wasn't sure where I was going, the
going itself was important to me. How I got there
was irrelevant, as long as I got there fast.

It is no surprise, then, that running became such a
big part of my life. Running suited my impatience. It
was the fastest way I could move my body through
space on the sheer raw power of my own energy. I
ran for almost two decades, until my knees and an-
kles started to wear out from the pounding and the
pain, until the well of my body's reserves ran dry.
When I stopped running, it was abruptly. I simply
could not push through another mile. I was lost for a
few years, without my runner's high, without my
speed, without my race.

In those transition years, I found my internal clock gearing down. I began to catch my breath. Unsure of what to do with the calmer pace I found myself in, I searched for other forms of distraction, other ways to fill the spaces in my life. So accustomed to looking ahead to where I thought I wanted to be, I ultimately began to look deeply at where I was. I found myself, with frightening revelation, standing still in the middle of my life.

Then, almost by accident or perhaps by design, I discovered walking. I had walked before, but only because I had to or because it was the most convenient way to get from one point to the other. But I had never really walked to enjoy walking. I thought it was something reserved for old age when running was no longer an option. When I finally gave in to walking as a legitimate, satisfying form of exercise and relaxation, I was stunned at how simple walking is and how it has always been available to me as such a perfect, easy solution.

All those years of running had taken me through city streets and down country roads countless times. But I really hadn't seen my world while I was running. I had been going too fast to see more than the most superficial details. Now, when I walk those same streets, I see things I never knew existed. I see the weathered fence boards, rusty gate latches, lazy lounging cats, gnarly tree trunks, and old buckets full of flowers that make up my neighborhood. I see the flushed faces of the children who play in the streets and feel the hot moist breath of the family dogs who come to greet me. I smell crocuses in the spring and moldy leaves in the winter. I watch the trees progress from first budding to frozen nakedness. I watch the grass poke up its timid green fingers in the spring and go quietly dormant in the fall. I witness the bathing rituals of sparrows underneath sprinklers. My feet have memorized the sidewalk cracks and curb cutouts. I see porch chairs and chimneys and brick retaining walls. I notice stone paths, mailboxes and woodpiles. I know the weathered roofs and sagging front steps of my neighborhood. I am part of it because I have slowed down enough to smell and feel and integrate it into my experience.

When I was running, only a part of me touched the earth, my heels or the balls of my feet grazing the ground every few feet with my long runner's stride. When I walk I am solidly in touch with the earth, landing full and square on my feet each step of the way. I am intimate with the bumps and cracks and slopes of my world. I know the crunching of leaves and pinecones underfoot, the splashing of rainwater on the toes of my shoes, the succulent cushioning of fresh fallen snow against my soles because my feet are completely grounded in them.

I am totally present in my world when I walk, fully immersed, my edges blending with the edges of everything around me so that I am no longer separate from them. When I walk, I belong. I am a creature of this world, no less than the sparrow or the lazy lounging cat. I am no longer fragmented, merely observing my world from the outside in. Instead I am dissolved into my environment like watercolors bleeding on a canvas.

The rhythm of my walking soothes me. The constant, cyclical movement of my body through space touches my deepest connection to all the rhythms of my life. There is something infinitely gratifying about ending my daily walk at the same point where it began. It completes my inner circle of mind, body and spirit. Walking has given all this to me. Now I walk because I can't imagine not walking. I walk because it is who I am. I walk because I must know my world by placing my feet in it, one after the other, until my journey is done.

Doing the Diva Dance

ANDREA KING COLLIER

Some people say walking should be used to make you more mindful and present. But when I walk, short of watching out for the dog with the angry drool or the car full of hormonally-challenged teenagers who take driver's ed at the high school next to my house, I am off on a real adventure. I am not trying to recapture lost days, remember my spirit, or thin my thighs for the new millennium. When I shoe up to put one foot in front of the other, I'm doing the diva dance.

Shortly after I started walking outside, I found that I could go farther and faster if I had music that had come to mean something to me, or artists that I loved. It gave me attitude. It gave me energy. It turned me into a diva. I wasn't walking, I was dancing and looking good doing it too.

Aretha Franklin singing "Freeway of Love in a Pink Cadillac," diva dances me past the tulips and irises. I have found that Mariah Carey is good for hills, and Gloria Estefan singing "Conga" is good for the home stretch. I cool down to Vanessa Williams singing "Save the Best for Last."

My diva dances are definitely girls days out. I made a few tapes with my favorite male singers, but find that when I diva danced with the girls, I become those women and they become me. So I stick to the ladies. And oh, what ladies they are. When I am diva dancing, I am Billie Holliday, with a beautiful gardenia in my ear. I am Janet Jackson singing about taking "Control" of my life and my hips. I am Diana Ross. I am Madonna.

I have to be careful sometimes. When I diva dance with Barbra Streisand, to "The Way We Were," I hit high notes that make the neighborhood cats wail. The dogs just run away. Until the neighbors got used to seeing me doing the diva dance, it was a bit off-putting. Every once in a while, other walkers cross the street to avoid me.

It is true that diva dancing can change you. When you do your thing to Tina Turner music it won't do to have on a pair of overworked leggings and a t-shirt that says "Sex Can Wait." So as I sing "What's Love Got to Do With It," I grow these fabulous legs—up to my neck, my walking shoes become serious Manolo Blanik stiletto mules, and I don a slinky, super short, yet simple sleeveless black sheath that shows those fabulous arms. The disaster concealed under my baseball cap becomes a fabulous head of hair, just made for shaking. Off I go, exaggerated strides, one long leg in front of the other.

Of course, forget getting your teenage daughter to diva dance with you. "Mom, what if somebody sees you doing that?" Or "Dad, can't you make her stop? She's ruining my reputation," she wails. She wants to know why I can't just walk around the block normally like other mothers. I happen to know that the other mothers are not having nearly as much fun as me.

There is a stale cliché that says music is the soundtrack of your life. When it comes to walking, it is true. By changing an ordinary walk into a diva dance your constitutional becomes a daily communion with the woman who never gets to come out and play. This diva inside you doesn't have to do laundry, or drive the car pool. This daily dose of Miss Thing lets you party in New York, be romanced in Miami, or sip Juleps in the South, instead of cut up a chicken for dinner in Michigan. Try it. Next time you go for a walk with your cassette, pass on Vivaldi, or the Gregorian Chant. Try a little "R-E-S-P-E-C-T," and do a little diva dance.

These Shoes Are Made for Walking

LAURA FASICK

Some people walk for their health. Some people walk to control weight. Some people walk for peace of mind. I have another reason: I walk in order to live up to my shoes.

No one who knew me when I was younger could ever have imagined that I would turn into a hopelessly addicted shoe-junkie. When fashion magazines gave lectures on matching shoes to outfits and calculating heel heights to complement hem lengths, I paid no heed. While my friends splurged first their allowances and later their paychecks on the most expensive sandals and pumps, I refused to even look at the word "shoe" in a sentence that didn't also include the word "sale." I bought paper-soled knock-offs at the cheapest discount outlets. Arch support, insoles, comfort, durability—what did those have to do with me or my shoes? It wasn't as though I had to *walk* in them.

My life changed when I moved from a big city with efficient public transit to a small town where cars provided almost the only means of transportation—apart from feet, of course. As a graduate student, I couldn't afford a car. But I still needed to get to classes, the grocery store, the laundromat, and a few other places not so essential but much more fun. Needing to walk, I did. I wasn't aware of how much I had increased my pedestrian activity until the day the sole fell off one of my shoes. I hobbled home, half-shod, half-barefoot, to check my other shoes. I realized why puddles seemed damper here than elsewhere: the soles of every pair of shoes I owned were worn so thin that ballet slippers would have been more substantial.

With the zeal of a convert I vowed that I would never go slipshod again—from now on my shoes were to be miracles of modern engineering and modern sport medicine combined: fit for an athlete! Heck, fit for an *Olympic* athlete!

In the years since, my shoe-passion has only grown more intense. Now at last I understand the glamour of footwear. Not of designer stilettos! Not of flower-trimmed sandals! But of shoes that render ordinary women into radiant-faced goddesses striding through redwood forests, able to walk forever. I don't imagine that a shoe will bring me a Prince Charming the way that a glass slipper did for Cinderella. No, instead I imagine that it will give me the energy and willpower to keep walking now that I do so out of choice rather than necessity. I buy shoes that are outrageously more athletic than I am. Waiting for an elevator, I'll glance at my feet, clad in gear suitable for scaling Mt. Everest, and I'll ask myself silently, "Are these the shoes of a woman who refuses to climb stairs?" As it turns out, sometimes they are. But more often, I'll climb. I'll walk to the library (ten blocks from where I live) in shoes designed for running marathons. But I will walk. Usually. After all, I have my shoes to live up to.

The Finish Line

June B. Lands

I am relieved to see the couple this morning as I walk across the sand to the water. They walk slowly, holding hands. He is trim, erect, with a graying beard and sandy hair. Her breezy lavender shirt and turquoise pants contrast vividly with her studied gait and bent form. I wave to them as I pass. I'm in the shallow water; they're a distance away on the firm sand.

Regular morning beach walkers know each other by face and form. If one does a no-show for a time, he or she's welcomed back with a friendlier greeting than usual. We're a motley bunch: the jogging couple with matching blue headsets; the pretty lady from the inn wearing a flower-covered hat; the woman running with her Dobie that carries a yellow plastic duck in its mouth. Most of us are out for body, mind, or spirit and have left self-consciousness in the closet with our winter clothes.

I walk the same stretch of beach every morning, with alternate days of weights and stretching. I'm not addicted; I'm afraid. I'm afraid I will outlive my body.

During my early years, I was plagued with thinness but blessed with a good frame. Even though I was not an athlete, I was athletic. I believe these things have held me in good stead while my shifting sands settled. Yet I'm afraid because I am predisposed to arthritis. When I look at my mother's swollen knees, when I see her strain to lift her body from a chair or take the stairs one step at a time, I want to run. But I know I no longer can run. And I cannot run away. So I walk in the water, forcing my legs against the water's resistance. I walk in the sand. I share my soul with the ocean and become momentary friends with people I don't know.

On my way back, I catch up with the couple. We walk and chat, and they invite me up to their porch for refreshments. The man helps the lady to her chair, offers me a seat, and excuses himself. When she lifts her head and smiles, I am surprised to see a face so youthful. With her white hair and bent body, and his erect figure and sandy hair, I'd thought they might be mother and son.

Over iced coffee, they tell me that when they retired, they began every day with a beach jog and finished with a game of tennis. Gradually arthritis began to steal her movement, bending her body so that she could not look straight ahead. She pats her husband's hand and smiles. I glimpse the woman she once was. She says that he is 72, that she is almost 10 years younger. A mental somersault tells me that she and I are almost the same age.

As I rise to leave, my knees snap, and my back reluctantly straightens with the rest of me. Heading south on the hard sand, I look back at the house and see the couple is gone. I start running, I run and run and run. I run down the beach and out to the street, all the way to my car, trying to reach the finish line ahead of arthritis.

Chariots of Lipstick

GENA ACOSTA

I stood at the bathroom mirror examining the shape of my legs. They looked pretty good, and I had done everything the books said: bought running shoes, socks, shorts, and even a vampy red lipstick to fit in the wee front pocket. I also got a facial. Finishing my leg examination, I nodded my approval. I felt ready for my first marathon. Unfortunately, no one else thought I was, because of one tiny thing. I don't run. Ever. I walk. Walking is good, walking is easy, and combining it with an event that killed its very first participant seemed sorta fun. So skipping all of that time-consuming training, I took my freshly facialed face and wicked new lipstick and went to walk the New York City Marathon.

It's wonderfully liberating to just show up at a possibly fatal event, and I, being free from all anxieties plaguing the people who knew what they were doing, was just ready to go. My only concern was to stay ahead of the sweeper trucks (the ominous vans that creep behind the last pathetic souls, ready to grind them into compost), so I expertly applied my lipstick and thought about what a hot little minx I would look like wearing my new medal. Then I was off.

The cheering crowds were tremendous. Herds of families, dogs, little grandmas, and grinning, clapping people who on any other day would look really evil screamed and yelled their encouragement. Balloons, banners, and thousands of colorful, mittened hands waved, making Brooklyn look like a shimmering rainbow. There was fevered activity in every inch of atmosphere. Runners dashed past me—bony runners, alarmingly fat runners, pretty runners, and runners who minced along as if they were holding in a giant fart. Then there were the runners who had stopped and were peeing. On everything. Bushes, curbs, walls, and police cars. No one seemed to care—least of all the two elderly ladies who were happily bouncing by in their matching, lacy purple bras, or the guy in the rhinoceros suit. The marathon is so fascinating when one is not busy doing all that dumb running.

Finally, 26 miles and seven and a half hours after I started, legs deliciously burning, I walked under the twinkling tree lights of Central Park. Briskly passing some runners who limped along like they'd been beaten with shovels, I was greeted by a cheering crowd of beautiful Wall Street banker men. All had brilliant smiles, radiant skin, and eyes yelling to me how good I looked. They yelled and screamed for me as if I were the finest athlete in the world.

And when I crossed that finish line, my soul glowing like the sun and feeling like the finest athlete in the world, I thanked God for my daily walks, facials, and pretty red lipstick.

Three on Loss

With Each Step I Take . . .

MARGARET BROWNLEY

Every death occurs in autumn, no matter what time of year it is, driving those left behind into the winter of the soul.

My own particular winter occurred after the death of my son. It was a long, hard darkness.

Somehow, I managed my normal daily walks because I feared if I stopped, I would lose what little control I had left. So I walked, day after day, week after week, each step cutting a new trail through the wintry terrain of grief.

Dr. Elisabeth Kübler-Ross identified five stages of loss and grief.

The first is denial. In it I wandered around the neighborhood in a daze, searching for my loved one. I knew he was gone, but my heart kept hoping that I would see my son drive by in his car, honking and waving at me, as he had done so many times before.

We walk with a rhythm unique to ourselves, a rhythm that matches the music of our souls. In those early days of grief, my inner music was slow and lumbering, but gradually the tempo increased. One day, I found myself walking fast, arms swinging. I became aware of my surroundings for the first time in weeks. This new awareness made me face an awful truth: my son was dead and he wasn't coming home.

I stopped in my tracks, unable to breathe. How could something so awful be possible?

My feet turned into mallets, pounding the pavement and driving me forward with fast hammering steps. Angry at the doctors, myself and even God, I broke into a run. I didn't know it then, but I had moved into the next stage of grief. It took weeks of fast walking to work through the anger and resume my normal pace.

I almost didn't make it through the third stage. Depression hit hard, driving me into a hole from which no escape seemed possible. For a time, I quit my walks; I could hardly get myself out of bed, let alone the door. The depression grew worse and out of desperation, I forced myself to walk again. On this walk I met a young child, bubbling over with excitement because it was his birthday. He smiled at me and I smiled back. It was the first time I had smiled in months.

I felt better after that little trek, and decided to walk again the next day and the next. If a short walk made me feel better, I reasoned, maybe a longer walk would take away the pain altogether. Two miles turned into five. Five into ten. I didn't know it at the time, but I had belly-flopped into the fourth stage—bargaining.

I wish I could say I moved from stage to stage in an orderly fashion. But long after grief was supposed to last, I found myself depressed again, angry again, hurting and crying again. We grieve in circles and spirals, sometimes going up, most often going down. But we walk in straight lines.

When others wanted to know after only a year why I wasn't over it yet, I walked. I walked on the day of my son's birthday, on the anniversary of his death, on that first awful Thanksgiving and Christmas. I walked in the early morning when sleep escaped me, at night with only the stars to guide me. I walked in desperate prayer and angry silence. I walked alone and with a loved one. I walked even when I was blinded by tears.

One day nearly two years after my son's death I stopped to stare at the rising sun—a golden spectacle that promised a beautiful day ahead.

Dr. Kübler-Ross called the fifth and final stage of grief acceptance. I prefer to call it hope. I will never fully recover from the loss of my son, but that morning new promise for the future burned a hole in the clouds. I felt God's comforting presence. I hurried home to tell my family how much I loved them. We planned a much-needed vacation—our first in more than two years.

I still walk daily and, on occasion, cry over my son's death. But more often than not, I smile because he lived.

"Spring" has arrived.

Running on Empty

ELIZABETH B. KRIEGER

When my world came crashing in around me, I hit the ground running. In the face of tragedy, I wound circles around the perimeter of our house, repeating to myself, Oh, my God . . . Oh, my God. Around and around I went, oddly consoled by this path of tightly spinning motion.

On that bright and warm morning, I was at home, painting my neatly filed nails, thinking about my date for the evening. My parents were serenely going about their day: Dad was mowing the mangy expanse of lawn, grown thick in the May sun, and Mom was watering droopy houseplants. My nails were almost fully set—perfectly splendid in Red Satin.

It was the morning I became an only child, the day a policeman came to our house. Somewhere, a few state lines away, the car my brother was driving had veered, rolled, crashed, and lay desperately still.

In the wake of that stillness, perhaps to keep it at bay, I had to move.

Movement came naturally to me: I was a gymnast until puberty, when I discovered tennis, making a name for myself as a little girl with a powerful racket. I'd always been good at performing alone, at pushing myself. When my brother died, though, I couldn't stop. A midsummer day became a chance to see if I could hack it in the heat and humidity. A winter date was a late-night run with a boyfriend followed by a frozen-nosed kiss goodnight. I took jaw-clenched laps around the neighborhood to ease the swell of a bruising day. I hated to sit idle, to torturously watch the numbers on a clock twist forward. No matter how much my body ached for the glorious torpor of a day's respite, I ran.

At college, I ran the campus until I mapped the curves of every soggy quad, every side street. I recognized city landmarks only as they passed at a dizzying, frenzied pace. I looked around less; I simply felt the well-worn comfort of unremitting movement, like a baby who can only get to sleep rocking.

It seemed like a positive thing. When I ran, I felt inspired. I brainstormed. In my head, I penned poems that would never make it to paper and rehearsed heartfelt apologies that I'd never deliver. When I stopped running, I was filled with awful loathing and cavernous grief. I'd feel my jaw tighten and my head grow leaden with anger. A vision of health in spandex and sweat, I was a mess.

Eventually, I outran my body and had to have back surgery. Once recovered, I scrambled back out there. I was hardly a stellar athlete anymore, just devoted to an intangible and lonely pursuit. I wanted to stop now, but I thought slowing down meant descending into mediocrity. I was running around with the joints of an old lady, the ego of a 16-year-old boy, and the issues of a troubled woman.

It's been a while now, but I have somehow stopped running. I am still active, but not in the same rough, thrashing way as before. I have slowed to a firm and blooming walk that speaks of warm, bright days and shiny lacquered nails. I've realized that this is not a sign of weakness, but the opposite. When Alex died, I couldn't face death head-on. So I tried to outrun it.

Today, I stride along next to the very questions and sorrows, many unanswerable and ugly, that had me running all along. Maybe I will never walk alone, entirely unfettered, but at least now I am walking wide awake, and I can see where I'm going.

An Unexpected Gift

RONNIE POLANECZKY

I quietly lock the front door behind me and inhale the early winter air. It has been over a week since my miscarriage, over a week since I've taken my regular walk along the river near my home, toward the chestnut tree that marks my turnaround spot. I dread this moment, but I can put it off no longer. I tighten the laces on my shoes and head south to the walking path.

For the past 10 years, I have walked this same route: some months, four times a week; other months, only once. There is another path, a more wooded one, on the other side of my neighborhood, and once in a while I venture there, drawn by the change in scenery. But I don't stay away long. I am a creature of habit, superstitious about toying with routine. I always return to the river.

Two months ago, when my pregnancy test turned positive, I fairly skipped along this path. Every bird looked wise, the river sentient, the river rocks ancient and solid. As I approached my chestnut tree, her muscled limbs stretched heavenward, I was acutely conscious of the new life within me. *Hello, tree. It's me. I'll be budding when you are; my fruit will drop when yours does. And then there will be a little one here with me. We are part of the same life force, you and I.* In that moment, I was struck by the simplicity and perfection of life giving birth to itself and at how, at long last, I was to be part of it. I felt at once newer than spring, older than time, larger than the body I inhabited, humbled by the responsibility that I carried.

Today, as I make my way to the river, I wish I had never experienced those feelings; now, along with mourning my lost pregnancy, I must also mourn the loss of feeling inextricably part of something larger than myself. My feelings are never so clear as when I walk this river path; the pain of awareness I've tried so hard to hold at bay these last days is hitting me hard. I quicken my stride, trying to alleviate it, but the intensity of feeling keeps pace. My breath is heaving, my heart is pounding, and, as I approach my tree, I realize I am crying—hard, loud sobs that struggle from deep inside and cannot be stopped, like birth itself. The pain overtakes me, blinds me, leaving me gasping and exhausted. And, like birth, it leaves me with a special gift.

For as I look at my tree, a voice speaks from deep within me, from within the force that gives the tree its strength, the river its current, the seasons their pulse. *Being pregnant did not connect you to the world's life force,* it says wisely, as soothing as a mother's caress. *It was a reminder that you are always connected.*

My knees weak, I lower myself to the frozen ground, hug my chest, and rock back and forth as grief gives way to relief. I lean into the tree's bosom, spent, as my gulps slowly dissolve into hiccups, then sighs. I wipe away my tears with the rough hem of my sweatshirt and quietly head back home.

No need to hurry now. No need at all.

A Good Walk Spoiled

Swept Off My Feet

EILEEN MITCHELL

I find it ironic that my podiatrist keeps WALKING MAGAZINE in her waiting room. Talk about salt in the wound! I'm not walking much these days. Instead, I'm visiting the podiatrist and the gym, thanks to plantar fasciitis, Latin for "royal pain in the arch."

That's why a shoe company's recent study of avid walkers caught my interest. The walkers had volunteered to give up the activity temporarily and track the physical and emotional changes they felt. The big news was just how dramatic those changes were, how much the women in the study needed walking for physical and mental balance. But it wasn't news to me. Ever since I started suffering from these foot migraines, I've known just how they felt.

The primary physical result of not walking, they said, was weight gain. Study participants complained that instead of compensating for not walking by eating less, they actually ate more, thus feeling sluggish and flabby.

No kidding. This inactivity is just what my fat gene has been waiting for. Helplessly, I've watched my thighs spread like the Continental Divide. My figure is now an hourglass with all the sand on the bottom.

That I anticipated.

What I didn't expect was how much I'd miss the other parts of walking—the sense of escape, the time to reflect, the simple joy of being outside. The study participants had said that for them, walking was holistic, as spiritually refreshing as it was physically stimulating. Amen. No matter how stressful the day or weary my body, once I kicked off those heels and donned my sneakers, my energy level made me Richard Simmons after a triple espresso. I pondered the day's events, revised a report, or relived a conversation. Maybe sang favorite songs from "Abbey Road."

Now, I'm a gym rat.

A gym, I've decided, is just an office where co-workers wear spandex. It's just as stuffy, just as constrictive, just as hierarchical. Instead of birds chirping, I hear grunts and groans. My body is exercising, but my brain is as stimulated as when I stand at the copier inhaling toner. And without the flexibility of walking (another virtue the study participants had noted), I now have to schedule my exercise routine. Fight for parking. Wait for machines. Wipe off sweat—other people's sweat.

I miss just looking around—and so did the walkers in the study. They reported feeling more attached to their neighborhoods when they walk. Only by walking did I notice Mrs. Forsberg tending her roses; Muirwood Park crowded with children; the sunset across Lake Chabot. And the smells: freshly cut grass, hot asphalt, the neighbor's barbecue, chlorine from the community pool.

But there was one thing I did not have in common with the study participants. They were thankful for the experience, saying they had never realized just how important walking was to them. But after eight days, the study was over and they got to resume their cherished activity. Probably with spiffy new shoes.

Not me—not yet. There's the matter of a little surgery to take care of first. But I have December 24th circled in red on my calendar. That's the day I can resume walking after surgery. I'll lace up my new shoes (complete with orthotics) and go to see how Mrs. Forsberg's garden is doing. How fitting that it falls on Christmas.

I can't imagine a better gift.

The Slip

Joan Anderson

Black ice put a halt to my invincible spirit and frantic lifestyle. Never having been stopped by illness or accident before, I was utterly dumbfounded when my feet slid out from under me one cold January night and splat—I was rendered immobile in a friend's driveway.

"Are you all right?" she called from her front stoop.

"Not really," I answered feebly, acutely aware that I had no feeling in my left foot and that it was dangling precariously from my lower leg. Sprawled helplessly across a patch of ice, I gazed up at the starry sky and ran through a list of all the things I had planned for the next day, to say nothing of a book tour planned for the next month!

Within minutes an ambulance was backing into the driveway, its ominous lights disrupting the darkness and adding to my trepidation. For my entire life I had shunned doctors for fear they would find something wrong with me. Now the game was up. I'd been caught.

Two medics hopped out, looked at my deformed ankle, gathered me in their arms and gently placed me on a stretcher. Hmmm, this isn't too bad. I could get used to such gallant attention, I thought. But then the siren jarred me back to reality. I sunk into the stretcher, stared at the ceiling and pondered my fate. It wouldn't be hard to give up my independence for a time, and I could easily "get into" being waited on for a week or two. But what would become of my daily 4-mile walk—a ritual which had become as necessary as bread and water? Without it, my spirits would droop along with my flesh!

The emergency room buzzed with efficacious nurses, orderlies and technicians who eagerly probed and poked every part of my body, save my ankle. When they finally got around to X-raying that which was mangled, I heard a gasp! "Bio-mallealor fracture," the radiologist announced, shaking her head and gazing back at me with pity. It sounded grim enough that I didn't bother asking for an explanation. Surgery was surely the next step one of the nurses told me on the sly. "You'll be here for at least three days," she added.

I quickly popped the Percoset they had been offering me to dull the pain and succumbed—blithely signed consent forms, decided on general anesthetic over a spinal, and was cooperative, polite and even trusting. I allowed myself one last stab of terror as they rolled me into the operating room, but a hastily made-up mantra helped calm my nerves and sent me to sleep: *It's only an injury, not a disease.*

Twelve hours later I awoke battered, bruised and with a Demerol-induced headache. I hurt too much to be kind to visitors or smile at the flowers that were lined up on my table. Furthermore, I was too nauseated to eat—a good thing actually, since I had become consumed with the fear of getting fat overnight without the benefit of exercise.

So far, nothing about this experience seemed encouraging or redeeming. But then my orthopedist appeared one morning and began raving about my bones. "Y'know I did an eighteen-year-old boy just before you. Your bones are every bit as good as his," he said. "It must be your walking regimen. All that weight-bearing exercise strengthens bones." (And this without taking hormones or calcium supplements, I thought smugly to myself.) His words rendered me measurably better. A few minutes later my confidence was further boosted by a nurse who took my pulse and declared, "You must be a runner. I can always tell because the pulse is nice and slow."

Two weeks have passed since that fateful night. I've graduated from a hard heavy cast to one that resembles an astronaut's moon boot, and I am into a period of forced relaxation which I hope will cast a serene look about my ordinarily harried face. I remember being overcome at the Madonna-like expression my best friend had after she broke her ankle and her family was forced to pick up the slack on all the household duties. When you are made to grapple with crutches, there is little else you can do with your hands. My days are spent luxuriating in bed until noon where I read, write and rest. Then I do leg lifts, buttock tucks and various upper body stretches. Walking has been replaced by a new exercise—an exercise in patience and trust. I am reminded of a line from Wendell Berry's aptly titled poem, "The Slip." "Seed will sprout in the scar." I await the mend and bless the regenerative powers of bones, never again to take for granted my precious ability to walk and then walk again.

Mid-Life Mileposts

MELINDA BERGMAN BURGENER

O ne month after his forty-ninth birthday, my
formerly sedentary spouse, Arnold the architect, left home and wife for a 212-mile solo trek
along the John Muir Trail in the High Sierra. This allowed me—a New Yorker by birth and a San Fran-
ciscan by choice—eighteen days and lonely nights to
contemplate a bout of absurd side-tracking I had
suffered seventeen years before; my own wilderness
experience.

I had just turned thirty-one, not a young age to
take up the outdoor life. In my right mind I would
have laughed in my own face. But my heart had been
snared by a full-bearded Wyoming mountain
man (who ordered his clothing from an L. L. Bean
catalogue and was raising two kids in an electricity-
challenged log cabin in the woods), and I was
hornswoggled. The family troika insisted on becoming a foursome for their annual spring-break back-
packing excursion. Montana's Beartooth Mountains
had already been chosen. Despite the ominous-
sounding destination, they convinced me—a wary,
bookish woman who had always opted for asphalt
under her shoes—that I could carry my pack, avoid
large carnivores and read my beloved Charles Dick-

ens in some coffee table–picture book paradise. Dickens would have encouraged me, I believed, since he was, himself, a great walker. Love and misinformation fogged my brain. I agreed to go.

From the beginning, I was deceived. Starting with the backpack. In over three decades on the planet, I had never heaved anything so heavy onto my person. Within forty minutes of slogging through boggy muck and up perpendicular ruts, I lost sight of Daniel Boone and his offspring. The speck growing larger on a distant snowfield eventually turned into eight-year-old Sylvano who had been dispatched to shoulder my burden so I could attempt to keep up.

We stopped wading through mud and snow at midday to consume a gaggly meal of cheesefood, nut butter and rice cakes; treats which caused my young cohorts to chirp with gourmandise delight. An hour after the feast, my mood was as foul as my digestion; and I sensed danger.

Although I was both wimp and neophyte of the group, I was also its sole member addicted to The Discovery Channel; I had a couch-potato's instinct for wilderness trouble. Even without suspense-building music, I recognized a bear hangout when I hiked into one. I whispered my premonition to Davy Crockett and Company, but was roundly pooh-poohed. Each assured me that although thousands of outdoorsy-types came to these mountains hoping to see bears, hardly anyone ever did, present bear-lovers fan club included. "You should be so lucky" were little Helen's words. Moments later, I was.

When that big mother emerged crashing through the brush on our left, we caught her gaze, turned and look straight up, above our heads, to the right. Two frightened fluffy cubs were hugging a tree, watching her, awaiting orders. Seven startled beings sharing a frozen nanosecond. I didn't enjoy a "told you so." My knees turned to marmalade and I tumbled backwards, down most of what I'd just climbed up. I couldn't help noticing as I rolled by my companions: their stunned expressions were no more beatific than my own. I vowed if I regained my limbs and lived through the next few days, I'd never go outdoors again.

So I left the mountains to the mountain man, returned to the city and met and married the architect, my perfect mate. He was skinny, beardless and obsessively attached to his work, which was done on a computer, which was plugged into the wall. This man was going nowhere near bears, nettles, nor backpacks.

I was deceived again.

The change in Arnold wasn't capricious; he didn't wake up one morning, declare he felt like a bit of exercise and take off for a 212-mile stroll. The High Sierra and declining muscle tone had peppered his conversation for months. Unfortunately, I was oblivious to mountain-man rumblings from reliably sedentary spouses and missed nipping it in the bud.

By the time my bearded, depressingly robust husband had finished hiking one-fifth the length of California, I was prepared to give up my seventeen-year-old vow rather than find myself filed under fungible on his computer.

So, one week after his return, I arranged an overnight stay for the two of us at a hike-in campground in Point Reyes National Seashore, a reputedly gorgeous spot, noted for its lack of bears. I borrowed a small pack, filled it with real food, gave all my other stuff to Arnold to carry and began to practice going without sleep.

My pack was just eleven pounds, my boots—worn only in Montana seventeen years before—were still comfy, and the autumn air smelled of spicy leaves and happy possibilities. We hiked six miles along the coast and through the woodlands; gentle countryside, so different from those craggy Beartooths of long ago.

We set up camp, enjoyed a fine dinner, then watched from a promontory as two bold fastidious gray foxes made off with our washcloths and the Dr. Bronner's Peppermint Soap we'd left on the picnic table. How sweet, how positively Walt Disney life in the woods could be! I fell fast asleep.

Around midnight, close-range hammering and strange guttural sounds entered my dreams and curdled my blood. Even Arnold awoke. He decoded the noise into tent-peg pounding and loud Europeans. Four Germans, believing their assigned site number to be the same as ours, tried to erect their tent on top of us in the almost empty campground. Arnold sent the confused tourists elsewhere, but my rest was finished for the night. So I know that it was exactly two hours later when some fierce, immense-sounding creature succeeded in mutilating what tiny peace of mind I had left. It rhythmically scratched and dug right under our tent for endless minutes while I held my breath, doing an involuntary charade for *paralyzed with fear.* We watched as it emerged at our feet, inside the tent—tall and shrouded like a ghost in our ground cloth. Its black and white tail gave it away just outside the screened flap. Carefully, we moved our tent off the skunk hole at 3 a.m.

After that, I did not attempt sleep. Instead—with a flashlight—while Arnold snored loudly beside me, I read.

Sunday morning, miserable, but fueled by infallible middle-of-the-night logic, I seized my opportunity to chat up my contubernal. Surely, an architect—of all people—saw clearly the folly of carrying his home on his back, only to set it down in a hellish plague of Teutonic tourists and smelly rodents. Convinced we were of one mind, I urged forward the plan I'd hatched for spending his next birthday in comfort and in France—my favorite place. We'd drive through the countryside in an old 2CV—Arnold's favorite car—with the window flaps pushed wide open and the sardine-can top rolled back. "*Voilà!* All the fresh air we'll need," I whispered.

I convinced him, easily, I thought, of the suitability of turning fifty in the place that invented champagne. Perhaps both delighted and surprised by my achievement—that I *could* keep apace in the out-of-doors—he listened with approbation and agreed. "Yes," he said, "yes, we're ready for France." Good as his word, Arnold enrolled in *French for Travelers* in night school and began hanging out at my favorite travel bookstore on weekends. Visions of luxe (Plumbing! Beds! Simmered foods!) danced in my head as I imagined our Gallic celebration of his half-century mark.

Three weeks ago, he asked me the French word for backpack; "*Sac à dos*," I said, thinking him generally wonderful, as always, for thoroughly exploring his new interest. Did he plan to regale French folks with our Point Reyes anecdotes? Then, last week he bought me a present; a book he'd discovered in *my* bookstore. I unwrapped it, all anticipation: Proust? Michelin Red Guide? An encyclopedia of French cheeses?

What I unwrapped was *Miles Away—A Walk Across France* by a deranged person called Miles Morland, who drew a line across France and set out with his wife, on foot, to follow it.

I figure marriage is a compromise. And it is, after all, Arnold's birthday. So, once again, we're taking off. This time, with *sac à dos* and many more mile-posts ahead than I'd bargained for.

Mondo Walking

The Shoes of Kilimanjaro

Cameron M. Burns

"There, ahead, all he could see, as wide as all the world, great, high, and unbelievably white in the sun, was the square top of Kilimanjaro."
—Ernest Hemingway,
The Snows of Kilimanjaro

I f you ever get to the foot of Kilimanjaro in East Africa, there are two sights that will take your breath away.

First is the mountain itself.

The looming hulk of this huge, seemingly out-of-place extinct volcano hovers above the East African plains like a gigantic, otherworldly spacecraft, quietly poised to nab hundreds of unsuspecting humans for exotic experiments on the far side of the Universe.

The second sight that will take your breath away—and leave you simultaneously scratching your head—are the shoes worn by the locals.

That's right, the shoes.

I'm not talking about just any local, however, as there are tens of thousands of friendly Tanzanians inhabiting the surroundings of Kilimanjaro and who seem to have a fairly normal range of footwear.

I'm talking about the shoes worn by the porters and guides on the mountain. They are, to put it mildly, the most astonishing thing you will ever see.

My odd relationship with Kilimanjaro's shoes began in late 1996, when I landed a job to write a climbing guide for an American publisher. My wife, Ann, was to accompany me on the trip, and, sometime around October, we began planning our mini-expedition.

Although Kilimanjaro requires little more than some steep hiking by its most popular routes, we took our planning seriously, as if we were mounting an assault on K2.

We assembled dozens and dozens of lists: lists of things to do, of people to call, of diseases one can catch. We also made lists of gear.

Nearly every item on our gear list was a simple matter of yes or no. Yes, we need it, no we don't. But things got awfully fuzzy when it came to footwear.

Would river rafting sandals or sneakers be better in the hot, dry towns? Would sneakers be adequate for walking through the jungles on the lower part of the mountain? Would I need plastic mountaineering boots at the top, or would leather boots suffice?

After much profound soul-searching, I packed up some sandals, a pair of sneakers, a pair of high-topped canvas boots, and a pair of mid-weight leather mountaineering boots. I also threw in a pair of down booties to wear around camp and in the tent. Once my pile of footgear was combined with

Ann's flotilla of sandals, boots and loafers, we had 12 pairs. *Enough* to make Imelda Marcos nervous.

At the airport, we paid $50 for our extra baggage (i.e. shoes), and once we landed in Nairobi, we had to tip taxi drivers and tour operators that little bit extra because we had so much stuff.

On January 2, our hired Land Rover dumped Ann and I, along with our guide and four porters at the Kilimanjaro National Park Gate. I was wearing my sandals and Ann had slipped on her walking shoes.

Our guide William wore a pair of crummy sneakers. They were at least six sizes too big and made him look like he was wearing clown shoes. I later learned they had been donated by a German tourist.

Our porters—Michael, Alan, Mohammed, and John—wore beach thongs. That's right, beach thongs.

Flip-flops. Sandals. Call 'em what you will, a flimsy piece of rubber about a quarter of an inch thick and held on by two thin strips of similar rubber running over the sides of the foot at an angle. About as sturdy as a cardboard box in a typhoon.

Regardless, none of the porters—nor William, for that matter—seemed the least big handicapped by their footwear.

Indeed, while Michael deftly maneuvered over slick wet tree roots with the precision of a ballerina, Ann and I tripped hither-thither. While Alan danced up short cliff bands scattered along the trail, we quavered in fright on the crumbling hand and footholds.

That evening, when we reached the camp, I exchanged my sandals for my camp booties. Ann put on some lightweight hiking boots. In the morning, I switched to sneakers, and Ann put on her walking shoes again.

As the days drifted by and we crept ever higher on the mountain, Ann and I changed shoes every half day or so. Sneakers to canvas boots. Canvas boots to walking shoes. Sneakers to leather mountaineering boots. Leather mountaineering boots to canvas boots. And so on.

As we fussed over our feet, our Tanzanian friends watched in amusement. We were obviously appeasing some strange Western deity who had bestowed some painstaking rules regarding feet.

On January 4, we reached the highest camp on the mountain, and finally the porters changed *their* footgear.

Michael put on a pair of penny loafers. The seams were split and resewn with white string. The soles were slick as ice. Alan and Mohammed both donned ripped sneakers, with treads more suited to a basketball court than a rocky trail. And John put on a pair of worn leather wing-tips, the kind a bum in New York City's Bowery might wear.

We sat around a small fire that night eating, laughing and sipping mugs of tea. Secretly, we were regarding each other's feet.

In the morning Ann, William and I arose, and toiled up 5 kilometers of frozen gravel to the summit, where we ran smack into a crowd, all milling about in the dawn light and celebrating their few minutes of glory on top of Africa.

Three German tourists wearing huge, green neon Koflach plastic mountaineering boots stood side by side with local guides wearing leather street shoes. A British couple, in $300-a-pair leather hiking boots and gaiters, slapped the back of a Tanzanian porter wearing a pair of lightweight vinyl cross-country skiing shoes.

We descended back to camp, packed up, and then turned our attention to the descent through the forests. Our mini-expedition was an enormous success, and we were ready to celebrate our incredible, historic achievement—even though we were just three of 70 who summited that day.

In 1968, two one-legged Austrians, Otto Umlauf and Thomas Karcher, who were crippled during World War II, climbed Kilimanjaro. In February 1969, seven blind African boys climbed Kibo as far as Gillman's Point. In 1994, American climbers Kevin Cooney and John Winsor ran up the Marangu Route, taking 7 hours and 11 minutes from the gate to the summit of Kibo, and 12 hours 45 minutes for the whole trip. And in 1981, Swiss mountaineer Fritz Lortscher reported that he had climbed Kilimanjaro at least 33 times.

These achievements seem small when one considers that many of the guides and porters have not only climbed the mountain over 200 times, but they've done it in shower shoes.

And here is the kicker:

A few days after our first ascent of the mountain, Ann and I bumped into Mohammed on the streets of Moshi, the small town sitting at the base of the mountain. He was with a group of fellow locals, all vying for a job portering for the next round of tourists.

And, he was wearing very nice, very new hiking boots, a far cry from the beach thongs and crummy sneakers he'd worn on the mountain. Ann and I took him aside, and tried to politely grill him about his footwear.

"These?" he asked in response to our accusatory fingers. "These are my good shoes. I wouldn't want to take them up on the mountain. I wouldn't want to ruin them. I use my old shoes up there, where it doesn't matter if they get damaged."

As I watched Mohammed walk back across the street to rejoin the group of porters, something similar to what Ernest Hemingway wrote 60 years ago in *The Snows of Kilimanjaro* came to mind.

"There, ahead, all he could see, as crappy as any product in all the world, tragic, worthless, and unbelievably flimsy on the trail, were the shoes of Kilimanjaro."

These Shoes Weren't Made for Walking

MARGIE GOLDSMITH

I often travel to exotic places for my work and have a "travel drawer" so I won't forget the important things when I have to pack in a hurry. Included is my passport, a travel converter with various plugs for different countries, a double voltage hair dryer, sneakers for walking, and an additional pair of worn-out walking sneakers. I take the latter as currency, not for working out.

Trading my sneakers started years ago, in Port au Prince, Haiti. I had stopped to look at some colorful street art. One painting in particular caught my eye: a primitive oil painting with tigers, zebras, and giraffes in a lush jungle, surrounded by green volcanic hills. I could already picture it on my wall, but the price tag was twenty dollars and I had no money on me. The artist was equally disappointed. Then he stared at my feet and brightened.

"I'll trade you my painting for those," he said.

At first I didn't understand. Then I realized he wanted my sneakers. "Wait a minute," I said. "You want to *trade* your painting for my shoes?"

He nodded.

I knew I could easily replace my sneakers but I'd never see another painting like this. It sounded like a perfect swap, and I convinced myself that if Peter Minuit could trade Manhattan for twenty-four dollars worth of trinkets, I could trade my shoes for a piece of art. I took them off as he rolled up the canvas. From his grin I could tell he thought he got the better deal, but I knew I had. I walked back to the hotel in my socks, happily carrying my painting.

Armed with the knowledge that used sneakers were a commodity, on a trip to Acapulco, I went prepared. When shopping, I walked around wearing a pair of worn leather sneakers with a pair of flip-flops tucked into my bag. One morning while browsing at a Mexican jewelry stall, I spotted a sterling silver bracelet inlaid with a star and moon motif. It was unique.

I slipped the bracelet on my wrist. It fit perfectly. "How much?" I asked.

"Thirty dollars," he said.

I wanted the bracelet, but didn't want to pay thirty dollars. I glanced around to make sure no one was watching, pointed to my sneakers, then looked at his enormous feet. I whispered conspiratorially. "I'll swap you for the bracelet. They're real leather and they'll be perfect for your wife or daughter."

He stooped down and examined my sneakers. "You give me these and twenty dollars," he said.

"These and ten dollars," I said.

He shook his head and I walked away, pretending to leave. I planned to wait a few minutes, come back, and give him twenty plus the sneakers. But before that happened he ran up, tapped me on the arm, and acquiesced. "Okay, Lady, ten dollars and the shoes." He snapped the silver bracelet onto my wrist. I was elated! Now I was not only the proud owner of a one-of-a-kind bracelet, but had also learned how to bargain!

It doesn't always work the way you expect it to. While in New Delhi, India, I saw an extraordinary wall hanging of Krishna and his maidens surrounded by sacred cows. I'd seen similar paintings, known as Pichwais, in New York, but they cost well over a thousand dollars. This was only one hundred. I was willing to pay the price but hadn't lugged my old walking shoes halfway around the globe just to bring them back home again.

"I'll give you seventy dollars plus these sneakers," I said.

He looked at my shoes, then scrutinized everything I was wearing. Suddenly his eyes lit up.

"I take your watch also."

The watch was a gift and though not particularly expensive, I had no intention of parting with it. I shook my head.

"This is a very fine Pichwai. You give your shoes, your watch, and seventy dollars."

"I'm not selling my watch."

"Then one hundred dollars," he said. "*And* the shoes."

"That's ridiculous! It cost one hundred dollars *before* I offered my sneakers!"

We finally agreed on ninety dollars and my sneakers. I walked off with my purchase, grinning in the knowledge that I'd made a very fair trade.

But I'm not in "international trade" merely to make a profit. On a trip to the Cloud Forest in Peru, I slogged in mud, hacked through the jungle, and climbed high mountain passes for a story. A pony carried my duffel bag, inside of which was a pair of worn walking shoes. At the start of the expedition, I'd decided to swap them for a maroon hand-woven poncho one of the horsemen wore. That night at dinner, the temperature was below freezing. I noticed the horseman was wearing thin cotton pants, no socks, and threadbare sandals which had been made from a rubber tire. His small gaunt frame shivered beneath his woolen poncho. I went to my tent, came back with the sneakers, and held them out to him.

"These are for you," I said. "A gift."

His face lit up as he took the shoes and then grinned at me through an almost toothless mouth. It was the best trade I ever made.

Frequent Flyer Walker

ANN HOOD

From 1979 to 1986 I walked a million miles. But unlike the religious pilgrims who follow Saint Patrick's route across Ireland, or the adventurers who walk across Nepal, I did not receive salvation or redemption and my health did not benefit from my walking. In fact, I did not even get any fresh air. I walked a million miles inside an airplane. For sixty hours a month, every month for seven years, I walked. I was a flight attendant.

I could say I walked from New York City to Cairo. I could say I walked from San Francisco to Boston, or Paris to Zurich, or Miami to Pittsburgh and I would be telling you the truth. But that implies scenery. It implies sparkling blue oceans and snow-capped mountains and cathedrals and rivers and rolling hills, when all I saw while I walked were clouds out the Chicklet-shaped windows, a lot of darkness, and sometimes a sunrise. *If* I even looked out a window at all, which mostly I did not because I was so busy walking.

I did see a lot of movies without sound, Eddie Murphy on the wall ahead of me, his mouth contorted, his eyes rolling, as I walked through the airplane saying: "Chicken or beef? Chicken or beef?

Chicken or beef?" There are many movies that I have seen dozens of times but have never heard. They are so familiar that even now I could not stand to watch them, although sometimes I do wonder what sent entire 747s of passengers laughing so hard.

No doubt you have walked up and down the aisles of an airplane, even if you were only trying to get to the bathroom. But to walk them almost non-stop is a different matter. And to walk them almost non-stop in high heels is an experience that is hard to describe. At night, on layovers in various hotel rooms around the world, I would lie on the bed with my legs raised and my feet pressing against the wall. This helped a little. But then the next day it was back to the high heels and the walking.

Much of the time I pushed a very heavy cart while I walked. This cart was full of beverages and cups and a pot of hot coffee and a carafe of stale airplane water. Many times the aisles were full of passengers who needed to stand. "Behind you!" I'd say and instead of getting out of my way they would turn themselves sideways and I would have to squeeze past them. This often made them angry. Other times someone would have gone to the bathroom and they were now stuck behind me and my cart. This made them anxious. They were afraid they would not get their cocktail or that somehow, inexplicably, they would never be able to return to their seat. To calm them—and to get them out of my way—I rolled my heavy cart way up the aisle so they could sit down and then rolled it all the way back. As I zoomed past, passengers yelled drink orders at me. People were always thinking they weren't going to get served, that they were being neglected or forgotten. But there are two things flight attendants always do: they give passengers their drinks, and they smile even as people yell: "Hey! What about me! I want a Bloody Mary!"

The worst part about my walking wasn't the yelling or even the sore feet. The worst part was when I walked and saw a passenger with a particular look on her face—eyes wide and horrified, hands over mouth. This is the look of someone about to throw up. A good flight attendant sticks an airsick bag in her apron pocket to hand to the airsick person. An unprepared flight attendant gets thrown up on a lot. This is bad enough, but on a five-day trip, the only clean uniform piece a flight attendant has is a spare shirt. That blazer and skirt has to last for days of zigzagging the continent, no matter what has landed on it.

Some routes are better for walking than others. London is good. The passengers tend to stay in their seats. Mediterranean countries are bad. Italians and Spaniards and Portuguese like to stand in the aisles and talk, often while smoking. If you have never walked through a narrow aisle clogged with a dozen Italian men smoking non-filtered cigarettes then you have missed out on something. Even when I reprimanded them for being in the way and for smoking while standing in the aisle, even when I invoked the FCC safety regulations, they smiled and called me "Bella." It is hard to get angry at smiling Italian men, even if they are in the way.

On red-eye flights I walked less. The passengers slept, except on flights to San Francisco where passengers liked to stay up late and drink and talk, as if the airplane was a large flying bar. At night, the lights were kept low. The shades were drawn. When I did walk, I flashed my little regulation flashlight to make sure no one had died or was dying or needed a 7UP really badly. I liked walking best on these all-night flights. It was quiet. I could walk slowly, taking in the airplane smells of fuel and recycled air and spilled soda. The hum of the engines sounded like a lullaby instead of the harsh way they sounded during meal-time when everyone was always talking loudly. And even the nastiest passenger looks vulnerable and sweet while asleep.

It is true that I have not been a flight attendant for over twelve years now. But I remember how it felt to spend the good part of a day walking the aisles of various aircraft. I remember how much I enjoyed walking on Lockheed 1011s because they were so flight attendant friendly, with galleys and little cart locks everywhere. I remember the way small children used to look when I walked past them, awestruck by the snazzy Ralph Lauren uniform with the shiny wings pinned to the blazer. I remember walking down those aisles over and over, checking that seat belts were fastened, that tray tables were in their original upright and locked position, that carry-on bags were safely stowed. I remember the smiles of little old ladies and honeymoon couples and businessmen on their way home.

When I fly now, I remember all of these things with great fondness. I take my seat and fasten my own seat belt. Inevitably a flight attendant walks by, on her way to stow an oversized bag, or pick up extra meals. She walks fast and with purpose. Since I was a child I wanted to be a flight attendant, mesmerized by the way they looked and all the places I imagined they went. Watching one now from this vantage point, I am happy for my million miles. I open a book and settle in for my flight. I stay in my seat. Happily, I do not walk.

Contributors

Gena Acosta is a Los Angeles native with a Master's of Fine Arts Degree from Long Beach State and when she is not dodging earthquakes, silicone-enhanced movie stars and palm trees, she enjoys freelancing for such magazines as *Roads to Adventure, Westways, Pets: part of the family* and *L.A. Parent.* Gena plans to do the NYC Marathon again this year—only better prepared.

Joan Anderson began writing magazine articles some twenty years ago before turning to children's books. She has written over twenty children's books, several works of non-fiction, *Breaking the TV Habit* (Scribners) and *Getting Unplugged* (John Wiley and Sons) and her recent memoir, *A Year by the Sea—Thoughts of an Unfinished Woman* (Doubleday). She loves writing articles for *Walking* magazine.

Violeta Balhas lives in East Gippsland, Australia. She is a freelance writer, educator, and mother to three children who regularly accompany her on her walks. Her mother, Nelida, who features in "Just Walkin' in the Rain," died in March 1999. Violeta dedicates this piece to her.

Melinda Bergman Burgener is a writer who lives in San Francisco. Her essays have been published on Salon.com and in books, newspapers, and magazines throughout the country.

Scott Breeze is a writer and inmate at Correction Treatment Facility in Washington, D.C.

Margaret Brownley has published twenty novels, and writes for TV. She lives in Southern California with her husband, and is presently working on a non-fiction book on grief and healing.

Cameron M. Burns, born in 1965 in Australia, is a Basalt, Colorado-based writer, climbing guide, adventure traveler, photographer, and artist. He is the author of six climbing guides, two novels, and thousands of magazine and newspaper articles. His photographs have appeared in dozens of publications around the world. He recently began guiding specialized acclimatization ascents of Kilimanjaro.

John Burroughs (1837–1921), an American naturalist, was best known as a writer on outdoor life. This essay appeared in W. R. Browne's anthology *Joys of the Road* (Atlantic Monthly Press, 1923). Reprinted with permission.

Andrea King Collier is a writer of both fiction and nonfiction. She has just completed a book of essays on the writing life, called "Oh, My Dear Writer Chicks," and a novel, "Breakthrough Blackness." She lives in Lansing, Michigan, with her husband and two children.

Betsy Banks Epstein is a mother of three and a writer based in Cambridge, Massachusetts. Her work has appeared frequently in the *Boston Sunday Globe,* the *Burlington Free Press,* and the *Cambridge Chronicle,* as well as in *Booming* magazine and *Pandemonium,* an anthology of parental humor.

Kathryn Dawson has published autobiographical essays in *Newsweek on Campus, Guideposts* magazine, and *Exponent II.* She currently takes her walks around the block in Dublin, Ohio.

Bill Donahue has written for *The New Yorker, The New York Times Magazine, Double Take,* and *Outside,* for whom he is a correspondent. He lives in Portland, Oregon, with his daughter, Allie, now six.

Lynn Duryee is a Superior Court judge in San Rafael, California. Her first novel, *My Treehouse,* was published in 2000 by Huckleberry Press.

Laura Fasick has lived, walked, and written in Toronto, Ontario, and in Bloomington, Indiana. She now resides in Moorhead, Minnesota, where she teaches English at Moorhead State University.

Michael Finley lives, writes, and walks his dog in Saint Paul, Minnesota. He has written several books, including *The New Why Teams Don't Work* (Berrett-Koehler Publishers). For more of his writing, check out *www.mfinley.com.*

Tom Glick graduated in 1998 from Goshen College, a Mennonite liberal arts college in Indiana, where he majored in history and French. He has bicycled across the United States and currently works as a legal assistant at an immigration law firm in Washington, D.C.

Margie Goldsmith lives in New York City but travels the globe to write about her adventures. Her articles have appeared in *The New York Times, National Geographic Traveler, Travel Holiday, Walking,* and *Tennis.* Her novel, *Screw-Up,* was published by Berkley Press and her work is included in *In Search of Adventure: A Wild Travel Anthology.* Goldsmith is president and founder of MG Productions, a New York–based video company.

Bill Harley is recognized as one of America's finest performers for families. He is a singer/songwriter, storyteller, author, and playwright, who tours nationally as a solo artist as well as with his band. With eighteen recordings and four children's books to his credit, Bill's humorous, yet meaningful work has also appeared in *Walking Magazine, RI Monthly, The Horn Book Magazine* and *The Michigan Reading Journal.* The recipient of numerous national awards including two Grammy nominations, Bill is also a regular commentator on National Public Radio's "All Things Considered." He makes his home in Seekonk, Massachusetts, with his wife, Debbie Block, and two sons, Noah and Dylan.

Hank Herman, humor columnist for the *Westport News,* is also an author of children's fiction. His latest book, *Marked Man and Other Soccer Stories* (Roxbury Park), was published in March 2000. Herman lives with his wife and three sons in Westport, Connecticut.

Ann Hood is the author of the non-fiction book *Do Not Go Gentle* (Picador, 2000); seven novels including *Somewhere off the Coast of Maine, Waiting to Vanish, Three-Legged Horse, Something Blue, Places to Stay the Night, The Properties of Water,* and *Ruby*; and numerous short stories, essays, articles and reviews. She lives in Providence, Rhode Island.

Jeffrey R. Katz completed a career change in May 2000 by graduating from law school and now works in Boston. Happiest outdoors, he regularly enjoys long walks with his wife and two sons, ages three and seven. His next writing project is a children's book about a dragon.

Clint Kelly has published five adventure novels including *Deliver Us from Evil* and *The Power and the Glory*. He has also been published in numerous periodicals including *American History Illustrated* and

Family Circle. He is at work on a true adventure set in the North American wilderness.

Judith Kirkwood stretches her legs in her neighborhood in Madison, Wisconsin, but spends most of her time sitting cross-legged on her office chair writing articles and essays for inflight magazines for TWA, American, Delta, US Air, and Frontier, and for consumer publications like *National Geographic Traveler, Country Living,* and *Family Life.*

Elizabeth B. Krieger is a writer and editor in San Francisco. She is currently an associate editor at WebMD.com, specializing in women's health and sports and fitness. Her work has appeared in both print and online publications, including *Walking* magazine, *Health* magazine, Salon.com, Sherwire.com, and Citysearch.com.

June Bishop Lands is a member of River City Writers and NFL Writers. Her personal essays have been published in *Florida Times-Union, Christian Science Monitor,* and *Byline.* Another piece is forthcoming in *Modern Maturity.* She lives and writes in the Florida sunshine.

Jodi Rusch Leas is a freelance writer whose essays and feature articles have appeared in the *Milwaukee Journal Sentinel.* Prior to becoming a freelance writer, she worked as a public relations writer and editor. She holds a bachelor's degree in Mass Communication from the University of Wisconsin. She currently lives in Wauwatosa, Wisconsin, with her husband and two sons.

Paul Lingel is a freelance writer who manages a 7-Eleven convenience store in Trenton, N.J.

Holly Love (*hlove@ot.com*) used her University of Pennsylvania degree to program computers before becoming a writer, editor, and wedding soloist. Her editorial, humorous, and autobiographical essays appear in national magazines and newspapers (including the *Philadelphia Inquirer* and the *Pittsburgh Post-Gazette*) and in her regular *Main Line Times* column. She and pooch Scooby live in Havertown, Pennsylvania.

Gregory McNamee is the author of eighteen books, the most recent of which is *Blue Mountains Far Away: Journeys in to American Wilderness* (The Lyons Press, 2000). His work on environmental and literary subjects regularly appears in periodicals such as *Backpacker, Utne Reader,* and *The Bloomsbury Review.* He lives in Tucson, Arizona.

Jim Merritt's essays and articles have appeared in *The Nation, The New York Times* and *The Village Voice.* His fiction and poetry have been published in national magazines and in anthologies published by HarperSanFrancisco and Dutton. A frequent contributor to *Long Island Newsday,* he also writes questions for *The Long Island Challenge,* a New York–area cable television quiz show.

Tracey Minkin is a freelance writer living in Providence, Rhode Island, with her husband and two children. Her work has appeared in *Travel & Leisure, Men's Journal,* and *Outside.*

Eileen Mitchell (*Mitchei@msn.com*) is a freelance writer who lives in the San Francisco Bay area. She is happy to report that her surgery was a complete success and now, when she isn't tapping away at her keyboard, she can usually be found somewhere on a hiking trail.

Beth Mund lives in Bridgewater, New Jersey, and she works as a professional recruiter while pursuing interests as a freelance writer. She earned an M.A. in psychology from Nova University in 1992. She and her husband, Mitchel Mund, have a two-year-old daughter, Gabrielle Ivy, and are soon expecting their second child.

Vicki Noll is a school counselor, an avid walker, and a freelance writer. In addition to *Walking,* her work has appeared in *Slice of Life, Grit,* and *The School Counselor Journal.* Her regular walks supply her with a time of reflection that, combined with the love of her family, keeps her sane.

Sister Josephine Palmeri, MPF, is from Pittston, Pennsylvania, a small coal-mining town near Scranton, New Jersey. Raised without a car, she always walked everywhere. Helping teens for forty years, Sister now teaches Spanish at Villa Walsh Academy in New Jersey. She loves Scrabble, jokes, people, teaching, reading, and storytelling. Her work has appeared in *Catholic Digest, Walking, Albriclas,* and *Today's Catholic Teacher and Ambassador.*

Ronnie Polaneczky's writing has appeared in *Philadelphia Magazine, Redbook, Ladies' Home Journal,* and *Men's Health.* She is a columnist at *The Philadelphia Daily News.*

Faith Coley Salie is an actor and writer living in Santa Monica, California. She is a Rhodes Scholar who received her degrees from Harvard University and Magdalen College, Oxford University. She does her best reading on the treadmill and her best thinking on her walks.

Carolynne Scott is a freelance writer and the author of two books, *Country Roads: A Journey Through Rustic Alabama* and *The Great and the Burning Alike,* a collection of short stories. She teaches fiction writing for Special Studies at the University of Alabama at Birmingham, and does her rambling with Buddy in the Crestwood neighborhood.

Lynn Setzer, a member of the profession writing faculty at North Carolina State University, is author of *A Season on the Appalachian Trail* and *Great Adventures in North Carolina.* She also writes travel and general interest stories for regional newspapers and magazines, as well as consults with businesses about their technical writing and Web pages projects.

Suzanne Strempeck Shea is author of three novels, *Selling the Lite of Heaven, Hoppie Shoopi Donna* and *Lily of the Valley.* A former reporter for the *Springfield Union-News* and the *Providence Journal,* she also has written freelance for *Walking, Yankee, The Boston Globe Sunday Magazine,* and *The Philadelphia Inquirer Magazine.*

Ned Stuckey-French teaches at Florida State University. His essays and articles have appeared in *American Literature, The Missouri Review, The Iowa Review, Modern Fiction Studies,* and *culturefront* and been listed among the notable essays of the year in *Best American Essays, 1997.*

Jacqueline Tresl is a registered nurse and freelance writer from rural Ohio. Her first book, *Who Ever Heard of a Horse in the House?* has caught the fancy of Hollywood media. Jacqueline and her amazing horse Misha have appeared in *People* and on "Good Morning America."

David Updike is a freelance writer who lives in Massachusetts. He has written a children's book, *A Winter Journey* (Prentice-Hall, 1984), and short stories for *The New Yorker.*

Kathryn Wilkens is starting a new career as a free-lance writer after thirty years of teaching Spanish and English. She has published articles and essays in *The Los Angeles Times* and *Walking*. She and her husband reside in a house that was built in 1903 in an orange grove in Upland, California.

Brenda Williams has published articles and essays in *Cruising World, The American Kennel Club Gazette, Healthways, Sunshine, Alive!, Family Pet,* and *Arise* and has published poetry in anthologies including *Encore, Collage,* and the *National Poetry Press' College Poetry Review.* She is a rehabilitation counselor in Billings, Montana.